DR. EARL MINDELL'S

Natural

REMEDIES FOR 101 AILMENTS

DR. EARL MINDELL'S

Natural REMEDIES FOR 101 AILMENTS

EARL MINDELL
R.PH., PH.D.

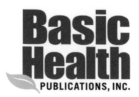

Basic Health
PUBLICATIONS, INC.

The information contained in this book is based upon the research and personal and professional experiences of the author. It is not intended as a substitute for consulting with your physician or other healthcare provider. Any attempt to diagnose and treat an illness should be done under the direction of a healthcare professional.

The publisher does not advocate the use of any particular healthcare protocol but believes the information in this book should be available to the public. The publisher and author are not responsible for any adverse effects or consequences resulting from the use of the suggestions, preparations, or procedures discussed in this book. Should the reader have any questions concerning the appropriateness of any procedures or preparation mentioned, the author and the publisher strongly suggest consulting a professional healthcare advisor.

Basic Health Publications, Inc.
8200 Boulevard East
North Bergen, NJ 07047
1-201-868-8336

Library of Congress Cataloging-in-Publication Data

Mindell, Earl.
[Natural remedies for 101 ailments]
  Dr. Earl Mindell's natural remedies for 101 ailments / Earl Mindell.
    p. cm.
  ISBN 1-59120-028-8
1. Naturopathy. 2. Dietary supplements. 3. Herbs—Therapeutic use.
4. Medicine, Popular. I. Title.
  RZ440.M5385   2002
  615.5'35—dc21

                                        2002007690

Editor: Carol Rosenberg
Typesetter: Gary A. Rosenberg
Cover design: Mike Stromberg

Printed in Canada

10 9 8 7 6 5 4 3 2 1

Contents

THERAPIES

Preface

Congratulations! By opening this book, you have taken a giant step toward better health and greater vitality for the rest of your life.

Because I am a pharmacist as well as a nutritionist and herbalist, I have a unique point of view on natural and alternative health. I have firsthand knowledge of how drugs work in the body, how they are prescribed, and why doctors prescribe them. I can tell you that the best thing you can do for your health is avoid prescription and over-the-counter drugs and turn to natural remedies to relieve whatever ails you.

The real secret to fabulous good health well into old age has a lot to do with common sense and moderation. If you put water in your car's gas tank, your car will break down. Doesn't it make sense that if you eat a lot of junk food and often drink sugary beverages that your body is going to break down? If you follow some very simple basic guidelines for a healthy lifestyle, you will find many of your chronic ailments vanishing. And you'll be surprised at how easy and how rewarding it is!

That's why I created my favorite natural remedies for 101 common ailments. These recipes will show you how your body can use all the wonderful natural remedies and preventive strategies to keep it running in top condition. I hope you turn to this book many times to find valuable information in your search for living a healthy and pain-free life.

Stay healthy!

Earl Mindell, R.Ph., Ph.D.

For a list of other books by Dr. Earl Mindell, visit http://www.DrEarlMindell.com.

Introduction

Natural Remedies for Your Medicine Cabinet

It wasn't so long ago that white willow bark was prescribed for pain, and chamomile tea for stomach aches. Today, herbal remedies such as these have completely disappeared from mainstream medicine. The pharmaceutical industry has learned how to take natural substances and transform their health-promoting constituents into synthetic versions, which have become our prescription and over-the-counter drugs. While these synthetic drugs have advanced medicine in some cases, they have done so with great expense, debilitating side effects, and interactive complications.

Lately, we've been relearning that Mother Nature really knows how to package remedies so that they are safe and effective. Once again, millions of people are turning to gentler yet effective means for curing all types of health conditions. This book features Dr. Mindell's favorite natural remedies for 101 common ailments. In these pages, this world-renowned health expert provides you with hundreds of natural time-tested remedies for whatever ails you.

Learn how you can use natural remedies to replace many of the most commonly used over-the-counter drugs in the treatment of the following ailments:

- Allergies
- Arthritis Pain
- Cardiovascular Disease
- Cholesterol
- Colds and Flu
- Depression
- Diabetes
- Headaches
- Indigestion
- Nausea
- Osteoporosis
- PMS
- Premature Aging
- Prostate Disorders
- Skin Problems
- Weight Loss

and more!

You'll find yourself turning to this book many times to find valuable information in your search for living a healthy, natural, and pain-free life.

A Note about Dosages

The dosage recommendations for the supplements and herbs listed in this book are for adults. For children between ages six and twelve, half of the adult dosage should be sufficient. For children under age six, always seek the guidance of a healthcare professional before administering any kind of supplement.

The herbs listed in this book can be taken in capsule form as directed on the label. When purchasing herbs in capsule form, look for the words "standardized herbal extract" on the label. Herbal teas are also available, but they are weaker than the standardized herbal extracts. Other herbal products should be used only topically. Their labels will state "for external use only."

The herbs and supplements recommended for each disorder can be taken together. In many cases, a remedy will have to be continued for at least thirty days before results are seen.

CAUTION: If you are pregnant or nursing, consult your healthcare professional before using any of these remedies.

Acne

Acne is an inflammatory skin disorder of the face, back, and chest. Although it is usually associated with hormone fluctuations during puberty, it can and does affect many adults. Whiteheads, blackheads, and pimples, which are characteristics of acne, result from an overgrowth of bacteria in oil-clogged pores. Although keeping the skin clean is very important in helping to control acne, it is not enough. Vitamins, minerals, and herbal supplements, as well as healthy eating and exercise habits, can be very beneficial.

SUPPLEMENTS

- Chromium: 200–600 mg daily.
- Selenium: 100–200 mcg daily.
- Vitamin A: 5,000–10,000 IU daily.
- Vitamin C: 500–1,000 mg with 500 mg of bioflavonoids daily.
- Vitamin E: 400–500 IU daily.
- Zinc: 15 mg of elemental zinc (read label), once or twice daily.

HERBS

- Echinacea: as directed on label.
- Goldenseal: as directed on label.

TRY

- Aerobic exercise.
- Detoxification (see TOXICITY on page 186).
- Drink six to eight glasses of pure water daily.
- Eat more raw vegetables.
- Eat yogurt with live cultures.

AVOID / WATCH OUT FOR

- High-fat foods and other junk foods.
- Refined carbohydrates.
- Stress.
- Sugar, caffeine, and chocolate.

ADD/ADHD

Attention deficit disorder (ADD) is a condition characterized by a short or poor attention span and inappropriate, impulsive behavior. Attention deficit hyperactivity disorder (ADHD) is ADD with hyperactivity. These disorders usually affect school-aged children, but may continue into adulthood. Symptoms include fidgeting, excessive talking, disregard of consequences, and an inability to concentrate. Psychostimulant drugs are often prescribed to control ADD/ADHD, but natural remedies, including nutritional supplements and exercise, offer nonprescription alternatives.

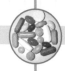

SUPPLEMENTS

- Calcium: 500–1,000 mg daily (older women: 1,500–2,000 mg).
- Magnesium: 250–500 mg daily.
- MSM: 1,000 mg, one to three times daily.

HERBS

- Bacopa extract: 100 mg daily.
- Club moss (Huperzine A): as directed on label.
- Ginkgo biloba extract: 60 mg, one to three times daily.
- Grape seed/green tea complex: 100 mg of each twice daily.
- Green tea extract: 100 mg, twice daily.
- Phosphatidylserine (PS): 300–600 mg daily.
- St. John's wort/phenol complex: 300 mg, once or twice daily.

TRY

- Allergy elimination diet.
- Biofeedback.
- Exercise regularly.

AVOID / WATCH OUT FOR

- Dairy products.
- Junk foods.
- Refined carbohydrates.
- Stress.

Alcohol Abuse/Alcoholism

An occasional alcoholic beverage is enjoyed by many adults. However, when indulging in alcohol becomes a frequent occurrence or when alcohol is consumed to excess even only occasionally, it constitutes alcohol abuse. Alcohol abuse can lead to alcoholism in susceptible people. Both alcohol abuse and alcoholism can interfere with work, relationships, and socialization. Willpower, along with natural remedies, can start anyone with this destructive problem on the road to sobriety.

SUPPLEMENTS

- Calcium: 500–1,000 mg daily (older women: 1,500–2,000 mg).
- Glutathione: 50 mg, one to three times daily.
- MSM: 1,000 mg, one to three times daily.
- Vitamin B complex: 25–50 mg daily.
- Vitamin B_1 (thiamin): 50–500 mg daily.
- Vitamin C: 500–1,000 mg daily.

HERBS

- Chamomile: as directed on label.
- Ginger root extract: as directed on label.
- Kudzu capsules: 500–1,500 mg daily.
- Milk thistle (silymarin) capsules: 140 mg, one to three times daily.
- Turmeric: as directed on label.

TRY

- Drink six to eight glasses of pure water daily.
- Drink a few cups of herbal tea, such as chamomile, throughout the day.

AVOID / WATCH OUT FOR

- Cough syrups that contain alcohol.
- Mouthwashes that contain alcohol.

Allergies to
Dust, Mold, and Dander

Allergic reactions are the immune system's response to perceived invaders in the body, such as mold or dust. These invaders, which are usually harmless, are known as allergens. An allergic reaction can range anywhere from mild to severe. Mild symptoms include itchy, watery eyes and sneezing. A severe reaction can affect respiratory and circulatory function. For mild cases and to reduce the frequency of attacks, nutritional supplements and other natural remedies can provide relief. See also HAY FEVER.

ALLERGIES TO DUST, MOLD, AND DANDER

SUPPLEMENTS

- Digestive enzymes: one to three capsules with each meal.
- Magnesium: 250–500 mg daily.
- MSM: 1,000 mg, one to three times daily.
- Omega-3 fatty acids (fish oil capsules): 50 mg, one to three times daily.
- Vitamin B complex: 25–50 mg daily.
- Vitamin C: 500–1,000 mg daily.
- Zinc: 15 mg of elemental zinc (read label), once or twice daily.

HERBS

- Borage oil: 500–1,000 mg daily (as capsules) *or* evening primrose oil: 500–1,000 mg daily (as capsules).
- Echinacea: as directed on label.
- Ginkgo biloba extract: 60 mg, one to three times daily.
- Grape seed extract (PCOs): 100 mg, one to three times daily.
- Licorice root: one to three 450-mg capsules daily.
- Quercetin: 400 mg before eating, one to three times daily.

TRY

- A colon-cleansing program.
- Detoxification (see TOXICITY on page 186).
- Drink six to eight glasses of pure water daily.
- Immune-system boosters (see IMMUNE SYSTEM, WEAKENED on page 114).

AVOID / WATCH OUT FOR

- Pets in bedroom.
- Excessive dust in bedroom.

Allergies to Food

A food allergy is an allergic reaction to a certain food, such as milk, shellfish, nuts, chocolate, or soy, or food additives, such as preservatives and colorings. Symptoms may include mild to severe skin rash, hives, gastrointestinal upset, and/or shortness of breath. Severe reactions can be life threatening. A person with a food allergy must eliminate the offending food from his or her diet, but may find natural remedies helpful in reducing the severity of symptoms in the event the food is accidentally consumed.

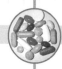

SUPPLEMENTS

- Digestive enzymes: one to three capsules with each meal.
- Glutamine: 50–150 mg daily.
- Magnesium: 250–500 mg daily.
- MSM: 1,000 mg, one to three times daily.
- Vitamin B complex: 25–50 mg daily.
- Zinc: 15 mg of elemental zinc (read label), once or twice daily.

HERBS

- Borage oil: 500–1,000 mg daily (as capsules) or evening primrose oil: 500–1,000 mg daily (as capsules).
- Goldenseal: as directed on label.
- Licorice root: one to three 450-mg capsules daily.

TRY

- Allergy elimination diet.
- Colon-cleansing program.
- Detoxification (see TOXICITY on page 186).
- Drink six to eight glasses of pure water daily.

AVOID / WATCH OUT FOR

- Excessive alcohol consumption.
- Food dyes, preservatives, and other additives.
- Foods known to cause an allergic reaction.
- Stress.

Alzheimer's Disease

Alzheimer's disease is the most common cause of dementia—a progressive decline in mental ability. It is often associated with old age, but can occur as early as middle age. The cause of Alzheimer's disease is unknown. Symptoms include loss of short-term memory, personality changes, and diminished ability to recognize people, places, and things. Although Alzheimer's disease is currently incurable, natural remedies can provide some benefit. See also MEMORY LOSS; SENILE DEMENTIA.

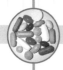

SUPPLEMENTS

- Coenzyme Q_{10}: 60 mg, one to three times daily.
- L-Carnitine: 50–500 mg daily.
- Magnesium: 250–500 mg daily.
- Melatonin: one to three 1-mg timed-release tablets before bedtime.
- Phosphatidylserine (PS): 300–600 mg daily.
- Pregnenolone: 10 mg daily.
- Vitamin B complex: 25–50 mg daily.
- Zinc: 15 mg of elemental zinc (read label), once or twice daily.

HERBS

- Bacopa extract: as directed on label.
- Club moss (Huperzine A): as directed on label.
- Ginkgo biloba extract: 60 mg, one to three times daily.
- Grape seed/green tea complex: 100 mg of each twice daily.

AVOID / WATCH OUT FOR

- Aluminum foil and cookware.

Anemia

In anemia, the number of red blood cells or the amount of hemoglobin (oxygen-carrying protein) in the red blood cells is inadequate for an ample supply of oxygen to reach the body systems. Common causes of anemia are excessive bleeding, decreased red blood cell production, and increased red blood cell destruction. Symptoms vary, but may include fatigue, weakness, and lightheadedness. Supplementing with certain vitamins, minerals, and herbs can aid the body's production of red blood cells.

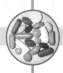

SUPPLEMENTS

- Folic acid: 400–800 mg daily.
- Iron (organic): 10–15 mg of essential iron daily.
- Vitamin B_{12}: 100–1,000 mcg daily.
- Vitamin C: 500–1,000 mg daily.

HERBS

- Chive: as directed on label.
- Dong quai: as directed on label.
- Quinoa: as directed on label.
- Rose hip: as directed on label.
- Watercress: as directed on label.

AVOID / WATCH OUT FOR

- Burdock root and yellow dock interfere with iron absorption.
- Excessive consumption of coffee and caffeinated soft drinks.
- Too much iron (that is, two to five times more than the RDA).

Angina

Angina is temporary pain or feeling of pressure in the chest due to a lack of adequate oxygen to the heart muscle. The most common cause of angina is coronary artery disease—a condition in which blood flow in the coronary artery is obstructed by fatty deposits. The pain or discomfort usually lasts for only a few minutes and is often triggered by physical activity. The underlying condition should be treated or, more preferably, prevented. Natural remedies, such as nutritional supplementation and certain lifestyle changes, can be helpful.

SUPPLEMENTS

- Carnitine: 50–500 mg daily.
- Coenzyme Q_{10}: 60 mg, one to three times daily.
- Magnesium: 250–500 mg daily.
- Soy isoflavonoids: 40–60 mg daily.
- Vitamin E: 400–500 IU daily.

HERBS

- Cayenne: as directed on label.
- Dandelion: as directed on label.
- Garlic: 500 mg daily.
- Ginseng: as directed on label.
- Hawthorne berries: as directed on label.

TRY

- Aerobic exercise.
- Eat fiber-rich foods.
- Eat foods that contain essential fatty acids.
- Eat more raw fruits and vegetables.
- Lose weight if necessary.

AVOID / WATCH OUT FOR

- Alcohol.
- All stimulants, including caffeine.
- Salt and sugar.
- Saturated fats.
- Smoking.
- Spicy foods and fried foods.
- Stress.

Anxiety

Everyone experiences some level of anxiety—as sense of apprehension or fear—at one time or another during the course of his or her life. It is a normal response to stress. Feelings of anxiety can range in intensity and can last for any length of time. An anxiety disorder is characterized by excessive, extreme, or unrealistic persistent worry about any number of things or activities. Certain herbs can reduce anxious feelings almost immediately. Other supplements and lifestyle changes can help, as well.

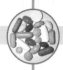

SUPPLEMENTS

- Calcium: 500–1,000 mg daily (older women: 1,500–2,000 mg).
- Inositol hexanicotinate (no-flush niacin): 250–500 mg daily.
- Magnesium: 250–500 mg daily.
- Multi–trace mineral formula: as directed on label.
- Vitamin B complex: 25–50 mg.
- Zinc: 15 mg of elemental zinc (read label), once or twice daily.

HERBS

- Chamomile: as directed on label.
- Hops: as directed on label.
- Kava: as directed on label.
- Skullcap: as directed on label.
- St. John's wort/phenol complex: 300 mg, once or twice daily.
- Valerian: as directed on label.

TRY

- Exercise regularly.
- Meditation and/or yoga.

AVOID / WATCH OUT FOR

- Aspartame.
- Caffeine.
- Monosodium glutamate (MSG).
- Refined carbohydrates.
- Stress.
- Sugar.

Appetite Loss

Any number of conditions can trigger a loss of appetite, including pinworms, gastrointestinal problems, tick bite, strep throat, hepatitis, and depression. It's a good idea to determine and treat the underlying cause whenever possible. Some nutritional supplements can stimulate the appetite, as can eating certain seeds and whole grains. Be aware that some prescription drugs can affect the sense of taste, which may result in a reluctance to eat. If this is the case, look into a natural alternative.

SUPPLEMENTS

- Biotin: 300 mcg daily.
- Calcium: 500–1,000 mg daily (older women: 1,500–2,000 mg).
- Copper: 2–3 mg daily.
- Magnesium: 250–500 mg daily.
- Vitamin A: 5,000–10,000 IU daily.
- Vitamin B complex: 25–50 mg daily.
- Vitamin B_1 (thiamin): 50–500 mg daily.
- Zinc: 15 mg of elemental zinc (read label), once or twice daily.

HERBS

- Black currant: drink as tea.
- Cayenne: as directed on label.
- Fennel: as directed on label.

TRY

- Eat more protein and whole grains.
- Eat pumpkin seeds and sunflower seeds.
- Sprinkle one tablespoon of brewer's yeast over food or dissolve in a beverage.

AVOID / WATCH OUT FOR

- Prescription drugs that can affect taste.

Arthritis

Arthritis is the inflammation of a joint or joints, usually accompanied by pain, restricted motion, warmth, and swelling. There are more than 200 causes of arthritis; rheumatoid arthritis and osteoarthritis are the most well known. Rheumatoid arthritis is an autoimmune disease that can affect anyone at any stage of life, while osteoarthritis is a degenerative disorder that is usually associated with advanced age. Certain nutritional supplements and herbs can help reduce joint inflammation, thereby easing the associated pain.

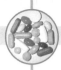

SUPPLEMENTS

- Bioflavonoids: 500 mg daily.
- Chondroitin sulfate: 1,000–2,000 mg daily.
- Digestive enzymes: one to three capsules with each meal.
- Glucosamine sulfate potassium: 700–1,050 mg daily.
- Omega-3 fatty acids (fish oil capsules): 50 mg, one to three times daily.

HERBS

- Cat's claw: as directed on label.
- Feverfew: as directed on label.
- Ginger extract (EV EXT 77): one to two 170-mg capsules daily.
- Ginseng: as directed on label.
- Licorice root: one to three 450-mg capsules daily.
- White willow bark: as directed on label.

TRY

- Acupressure.
- Detoxification (see TOXICITY on page 186).
- Exercise moderately.
- Yoga.

AVOID / WATCH OUT FOR

- Environmental toxins, including pesticides.
- Food allergies.
- Hydrogenated oils.
- Junk food and fatty, greasy foods.
- NSAIDs (nonsteroidal anti-inflammatory drugs), such as aspirin and ibuprofen.

Asthma

ASTHMA

In asthma, there is a widespread narrowing of the bronchial airways, which leads to coughing, wheezing, and difficulty breathing. In susceptible individuals, asthmatic reactions can be triggered by certain stimuli, such as exercise, cold air, and allergens, including pollen, animal dander, and dust mites. Stress and anxiety can also trigger an asthma attack. In some cases, this condition can be life threatening and should be treated accordingly. Natural remedies for asthma can help reduce the severity and frequency of attacks.

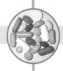

SUPPLEMENTS

- Magnesium: 250–500 mg daily.
- Multi–trace mineral formula: as directed on label.
- Vitamin B complex: 25–50 mg daily.
- Vitamin C: 500–1,000 mg with 500 mg of bioflavonoids daily.

HERBS

- Ephedra: as directed on label.
- Ginger extract (EV EXT 77): one to two 170-mg capsules daily.
- Ginseng: as directed on label.
- Licorice root: one to three 450-mg capsules daily.

TRY

- Acupuncture.
- Detoxification (see TOXICITY on page 186).
- Meditation and/or yoga.
- Immune-system boosters (see IMMUNE SYSTEM, WEAKENED on page 114).
- Use dust mite protectors and an air purifier in your home.

AVOID / WATCH OUT FOR

- Allergies to dust, pollen, mold, and dander.
- Leaky gut syndrome.
- Stress.
- Synthetic estrogens/progestins (birth control pills and HRT).

Athlete's Foot

Athlete's foot, also known as foot ringworm, is a common skin infection caused by fungi that thrive in the warm, moist areas between the toes. Symptoms can range from mild scaling to an itchy, painful rash, and in more severe cases, fluid-filled blisters. The infection can spread from the toes to the bottoms and sides of the feet. In addition to natural remedies, keeping the feet clean and dry and wearing shoes that allow the feet to breathe work well to clear up the infection and keep the risk of reinfection minimal. See also FUNGAL SKIN INFECTIONS.

SUPPLEMENTS

- MSM: 1,000 mg, one to three times daily.
- Probiotics: one to three capsules or one
  tablespoon of refrigerated liquid probiotics,
  up to three times daily before meals;
  or acidophilus: one to three (multi-billion
  count) capsules before meals.
- Vitamin B complex: 25–50 mg daily.
- Vitamin C: 500–1,000 mg daily.
- Zinc: 15 mg of elemental zinc (read label),
  once or twice daily.

HERBS

- Garlic: 500 mg daily.
- Tea tree oil: apply topically twice daily.

TRY

- Keep feet dry.
- Soak feet in mixture of vinegar and water.

AVOID / WATCH OUT FOR

- Bare feet in public locker rooms.
- Fried, greasy foods.
- Processed foods.
- Sugar and sugary beverages.

Backaches/Back Pain

Aches and pains in the back can be symptoms of any number of conditions, including muscle strain, injury, osteoarthritis, and pregnancy. Steps should be taken to determine the cause of the pain. If the cause of the pain is due to strain, injury, or overuse, resting, supplementing with nutrients and herbs, and trying alternative healthcare treatments, such as chiropractic, all can provide relief. Activities, such as lifting heavy boxes, should be avoided whenever possible; if necessary, however, proper lifting techniques can reduce the risk of injury or strain.

SUPPLEMENTS

- Calcium: 500–1,000 mg daily (older women: 1,500–2,000 mg).
- DLPA (dl-phenylalanine): 375 mg, one or two capsules every four hours for discomfort.
- Glucosamine sulfate potassium: 700–1,050 mg daily.
- Magnesium: 250–500 mg daily.
- Multi–trace mineral formula: as directed on label.

HERBS

- Feverfew: as directed on label.
- Kava: as directed on label.
- St. John's wort/phenol complex: 300 mg, once or twice daily.
- White willow bark: one to two 500-mg capsules, two to three times daily.

TRY

- Acupuncture.
- Chiropractic.
- Exercises for back and stomach muscles.
- Lose excess weight.
- Yoga.

AVOID / WATCH OUT FOR

- Constipation.
- Extra body weight.
- High heels.
- Improper lifting.
- Overdoing exercise.

Bad Breath (Halitosis)

Bad breath (halitosis) can be either a temporary or a chronic condition. Temporary bad breath can result from eating certain foods, such as onions or garlic; smoking; or taking certain prescription drugs. Chronic bad breath can have more serious causes, including tooth or gum disease, poor digestion, liver disease, and diabetes. Frequent proper brushing, including a light brushing of the tongue, and flossing are, of course, the first line of treatment. Nutritional supplements and other steps can be taken to reduce or eliminate unpleasant odor.

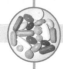

SUPPLEMENTS

- Acidophilus: one to three (multi-billion count) capsules before each meal.
- Betaine hydrochloride (HCL): one 150-mg capsule with each meal.
- Digestive enzymes: one to three capsules with each meal.
- Vitamin A: 5,000–10,000 IU daily.
- Vitamin B complex: 25–50 mg daily.
- Vitamin C: 500–1,000 mg daily.
- Zinc: 15 mg of elemental zinc (read label), once or twice daily.

HERBS

- Chlorophyll: as directed on label.
- Parsley: as directed on label.

TRY

- Detoxification (see TOXICITY on page 186).
- Drink six to eight glasses of pure water daily.
- Eat more fiber-rich foods.
- Eat more raw fruits and vegetables.
- Use dental floss.

AVOID / WATCH OUT FOR

- Mouthwash containing sugar, alcohol, and dyes.
- Offending foods.

Blood Pressure, High

The force that blood puts on the walls of the veins, arteries, and heart is known as blood pressure. High blood pressure, also called hypertension, is a condition in which the pressure is abnormally high. The cause of hypertension is unclear, and the condition can remain symptomless for years, increasing the risk of life-threatening conditions, such as heart attack, heart failure, and stroke. With proper care, including natural remedies, this condition can be controlled to prevent complications.

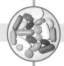

SUPPLEMENTS

- Coenzyme Q_{10}: 60 mg, one to three times daily.
- Magnesium: 250–500 mg daily.
- Vitamin E: 400–500 IU daily.

HERBS

- Garlic: 500 mg daily.
- Ginseng: as directed on label.
- Hawthorn berries: as directed on label.

TRY

- Eat six stalks of celery or the juice equivalent daily.
- Exercise regularly.
- Lose weight if necessary.
- Meditation and/or yoga.
- Reduce stress.

AVOID / WATCH OUT FOR

- Chronic stress.
- High-fat diet.
- Long-term supplementation of licorice with glycyrrhizin.
- Obesity.

Blood Sugar, High/Low

Blood sugar is the amount of glucose (a simple sugar) in the blood. It is normal for blood-sugar levels to vary throughout the day. However, levels that are chronically either too high or too low indicate an underlying condition, such as diabetes or hypoglycemia, respectively. Treating the underlying condition is paramount, but steps can be taken to stabilize blood sugar naturally.

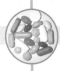

SUPPLEMENTS

- Chromium: 200–600 mg daily.
- Essential fatty acids capsules: 250 mg, one to three times daily.
- Inositol hexanicotinate (no-flush niacin): 250–500 mg daily.
- MSM: 1,000 mg, one to three times daily.
- Vanadium (Vanadyl): 10 mg daily.
- Vitamin C: 500–1,000 mg daily.
- Vitamin E: 400–500 IU daily.

HERBS

- Ginkgo biloba extract: 60 mg, one to three times daily.
- Ginseng: as directed on label.
- Grape seed extract (PCOs): 100 mg, one to three times daily.

TRY

- Eat more vegetables.
- Exercise.
- Lose weight if necessary.

AVOID / WATCH OUT FOR

- All sugars and refined carbohydrates.
- Excess carbohydrates.
- Processed foods.

Breast Cancer

Breast cancer is cancer of the breast tissue. It is classified by the type of tissue in which it originates, such as the milk ducts or connective tissue, and by how much it has spread. Symptoms that may indicate breast cancer include a lump in the breast, chronic swelling of the breast, and changes in shape of the breast or nipple. Treatment may involve surgery, chemotherapy, radiation therapy, and/or hormone-blocking drugs. Natural remedies may help delay or avoid the onset of breast cancer.

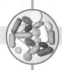

SUPPLEMENTS

- Flaxseed oil (refrigerated): 1 tsp of the oil; or one to three 500-mg capsules daily.
- Limonene: 5–50 mg daily.
- Melatonin: one 3-mg timed-release tablet one to two hours before bedtime.
- Selenium: 100–200 mcg daily.
- Soy isoflavonoids: 40–60 mg daily.

HERBS

- Psyllium: as directed on label.

TRY

- Drink soymilk and soy shakes.
- Eat soybeans.
- Eat wheat bran.

AVOID / WATCH OUT FOR

- High-fat foods.
- Low-fiber foods.
- Processed foods.

Bruises

Bruises form from breakages of small blood vessels in the skin. Blood leaks out of the damaged vessels, leaving red dots or bluish-purple marks that fade over time. It is normal for bruises to develop from a hard blow to the body; however, chronic bruising may indicate a problem with blood-clotting. Such a problem can be determined through blood tests. Bruises respond very well to natural therapies. Nutritional supplements and herbs applied topically can speed recovery time and help the bruise fade quickly.

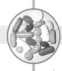

SUPPLEMENTS

- Coenzyme Q_{10}: 60 mg, one to three times daily.
- Digestive enzymes: one to three capsules with each meal.
- Rutin: 50 mg, one to three times daily.
- Vitamin A: 5,000–10,000 IU daily.
- Vitamin C: 500–1,000 mg with 500 mg of bioflavonoids daily.
- Vitamin E: 400–500 IU daily.

HERBS

- Aloe vera gel: apply topically as directed on label.
- Arnica homeopathic tablets: dissolve under tongue as directed on label.
- Calendula ointment or gel: apply topically as directed on label.
- Comfrey: apply topical preparation as directed on label.
- Garlic: 500 mg daily.
- White willow bark: one to two 500-mg capsules, two to three times daily.
- Witch hazel: apply topical preparation as directed on label.

TRY

- Apply an ice pack.
- Eat leafy green vegetables and fresh fruit, especially pineapple.
- Homeopathic bruise remedy.

AVOID / WATCH OUT FOR

- Taking aspirin in excess (more than six 325-mg tablets per day).

Burns

BURNS

Burns occur when the skin is exposed to high heat, certain chemicals, or intense electrical currents. Sometimes the underlying tissue and, in severe cases, the internal organs can be damaged. Burns range from first degree (the least severe) to third degree (the most severe). Minor burns respond well to home treatment; however, severe burns require immediate medical care. For minor burns and recovery from severe burns, natural remedies can provide much-needed relief and quicker healing.

SUPPLEMENTS

- Coenzyme Q_{10}: 60 mg, one to three times daily.
- MSM: 1,000 mg, one to three times daily.
- Potassium: 99 mg, one to three times daily.
- Selenium: 100–200 mcg daily.
- Vitamin A: 5,000–10,000 IU daily.
- Vitamin C: 500–1,000 mg daily.
- Vitamin E: 400–500 IU daily.
- Zinc: 15 mg of elemental zinc (read label), once or twice daily.

HERBS

- Aloe vera gel: apply topically as directed on label.

TRY

- Apply a cold compress to the burn.
- Drink eight to ten glasses of pure water daily.
- High-protein diet.
- Homeopathic burn remedy.
- Use a bacteria-killing spray.

AVOID / WATCH OUT FOR

- Do not apply any type of butter to the burn.
- Do not break blisters.

Cancer Prevention

Cancer is one of the most dreaded diseases. It results from abnormal, uncontrollable cell growth and can affect any tissue in the body. That's why there are so many different types of cancer. Both genetic and environmental factors can increase the risk of developing this often life-threatening disease. If you are at high risk, it would serve you well to follow a cancer-preventive daily regimen, including nutritional supplements and healthy foods, and to avoid cancer-causing substances, such as cigarette smoke and environmental toxins.

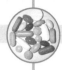

SUPPLEMENTS

- Cysteine: 100–250 mg, one to two times daily.
- Folic acid: 400–800 mg daily.
- Glutathione: 50 mg, one to three times daily.
- Manganese: 9 mg daily.
- Selenium: 100–200 mcg daily.
- Vitamin A: 5,000–10,000 IU daily.
- Vitamin B_6 (pyridoxine): 25–50 mg daily.
- Vitamin E: 400–500 IU daily.
- Zinc: 15 mg of elemental zinc (read label), once or twice daily.

HERBS

- Cat's claw: as directed on label.
- Garlic: 500 mg daily.
- Ginseng: as directed on label.
- Quercetin: 400 mg before eating, one to three times daily.

TRY

- Detoxification (see TOXICITY on page 186).
- Eat legumes/beans and soy products.
- Eat more fiber-rich foods.
- Eat more red, yellow, and orange fruits and vegetables.

AVOID / WATCH OUT FOR

- Emotional stress.
- Environmental toxins, such as pesticides and herbicides.
- Food additives.
- Radiation.
- Smoking.

Candidiasis

Candidiasis is a yeastlike fungal infection of the muscous membranes caused by the various strains of *Candida,* most usually *C. albicans.* Symptoms, such as white patches in the mouth or red skin lesions, vary depending on the infection site. Common sites include the mouth, vagina, respiratory tract, and the skin folds. In rare cases, it may spread throughout the body. Usually treated with anitfungal drugs, this condition responds well to natural remedies. See also FUNGAL SKIN INFECTIONS; VAGINAL YEAST INFECTIONS.

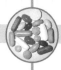

SUPPLEMENTS

- Digestive enzymes: one to three capsules with each meal.
- Essential fatty acids capsules: 250 mg, one to three times daily.
- MSM: 1,000 mg, one to three times daily.
- Multivitamin/mineral formula: as directed on label.
- Probiotics: one to three capsules or one tablespoon of refrigerated liquid probiotics, up to three times daily before meals; or acidophilus: one to three (multi-billion count) capsules before meals.
- Selenium: 100–200 mcg daily.

HERBS

- Garlic: 500 mg daily.

TRY

- Cleansing diet.
- Detoxification (see TOXICITY on page 186).
- Vinegar or yogurt douche.

AVOID / WATCH OUT FOR

- Alcohol, sugar, and yeast.
- Antibiotics and oral contraceptives.
- Chemical cleaners.
- Highly alkaline and acid foods.
- Mold.
- Mothballs.

Cardiovascular Disease

Cardiovascular disease is a catchall term for disorders of the heart and blood vessels, including heart attack, stroke, and heart failure. A properly functioning cardiovascular system is essential for the circulation of blood around the body. A block in the flow of blood anywhere in the body can have devastating effects. Therefore, preventing and controlling this disease is extremely important. There are many natural steps a person can take to manage an existing cardiovascular condition, including taking supplements and making important lifestyle changes. See also STROKE.

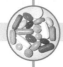

SUPPLEMENTS

- Coenzyme Q_{10}: 60 mg, one to three times daily.
- Cysteine: 100–250 mg, one to two times daily
- Glutathione: 50 mg, one to three times daily.
- Magnesium: 250–500 mg daily.
- Selenium: 100–200 mcg daily.
- Vitamin B complex: 25–50 mg daily.
- Vitamin C: 500–1,000 mg daily.
- Vitamin E: 400–500 IU daily.

HERBS

- Cayenne: as directed on label.
- Garlic: 500 mg daily.
- Ginseng: as directed on label.
- Hawthorn berries: as directed on label.

TRY

- Drink red wine.
- Eat high-fiber foods and soy products.
- Eat less red meat and more fish.
- Eat more vegetables and fruit.
- Exercise regularly.
- Lose weight if necessary.
- Reduce dietary fat.

AVOID / WATCH OUT FOR

- Processed foods.
- Refined and hydrogenated oils.
- Salt and sugar.
- Smoking.
- Stress.
- Too much coffee and tea (more than three cups daily).

Carpal Tunnel Syndrome

Carpal tunnel syndrome is a relatively common condition of one or both hands resulting from compression of the nerve that travels through the wrist. Repetitive movements of the hands, such as typing or using a screwdriver, have been implicated as a cause. Symptoms include numbness, tingling, and pain, sometimes traveling up to the arms and shoulders. Avoiding aggravating positions, along with taking nutritional supplements, can often provide relief.

SUPPLEMENTS

- MSM: 1,000 mg, one to three times daily.
- Vitamin B complex: 25–50 mg daily.
- Vitamin B_6 (pyridoxine): 25–50 mg daily.

HERBS

- No herbs apply.

TRY

- Stretch the hands, wrists, arms, and shoulders every fifteen minutes.
- Massage.
- Move keyboard to a different position.
- Slope chair slightly forward.

AVOID / WATCH OUT FOR

- Repetitive motions.
- Sitting in same position for long periods.

Cataracts

A cataract is an opacity, or clouding, of the
eye's lens. The clouding results in blurred vision,
which progressively worsens, leading to blindness. This condition is most commonly seen in
people of advanced age, but may occur earlier
in its congenital form or as a complication of
other diseases, such as diabetes. A cataract
will not improve on its own, and surgery may
become necessary to restore sight. However,
the progression may be slowed by taking
nutritional supplements and by following
some commonsense advice. See also
VISION PROBLEMS.

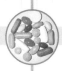

SUPPLEMENTS

- Beta-carotene: 10,000–20,000 IU daily.
- Glutathione: 50 mg, one to three times daily.
- Lutein: 6–20 mg daily.
- Multivitamin/mineral/antioxidant formula: as directed on label.
- Quercetin: 400 mg before eating, one to three times daily.
- Riboflavin (vitamin B$_2$): 50–100 mg daily.
- Vitamin C: 500–1,000 mg daily.
- Vitamin E: 400–500 IU daily.
- Zeaxanthin: 30–130 mg daily.

HERBS

- Amalaki: as directed on label.
- Bilberry extract: as directed on label.
- Marigold: as directed on label.

TRY

- Eat more fresh fruits and vegetables.
- Wear good quality sunglasses with UV-ray protection.

AVOID / WATCH OUT FOR

- Direct exposure to sunlight for long periods.
- Smoking.

Cervical Cancer

Cancer of the cervix—the outer edge of the uterus—is one of the more common cancers of the female reproductive system. Women between the ages of thirty-five and fifty-five are most often affected. Often symptomless until the late stages of the disease, cervical cancer usually can be detected by a Pap test. Taking nutritional supplements and making simple lifestyle changes can reduce the risk of this type of cancer, and can only benefit those who have it. See also CANCER PREVENTION.

CERVICAL CANCER

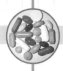

SUPPLEMENTS

- Folic acid: 400–800 mg daily.
- Lycopene: 6–10 mg daily.
- Vitamin B_{12}: 100–1,000 mcg daily.

HERBS

- No herbs apply.

TRY

- Eat more tomatoes, citrus fruits, whole grains, yeast, liver, and dark green vegetables.

AVOID / WATCH OUT FOR

- Many sexual partners.
- Smoking.

Cholesterol, Elevated

Cholesterol is one of the two major fats found in the blood. While the body needs this fat to perform certain functions, too much of the "bad" type (LDL cholesterol) circulating in the bloodstream can contribute to problems such as heart disease. Several factors can increase cholesterol levels, including diabetes, a diet high in saturated fats, and heredity. Fortunately, elevated cholesterol levels respond well to nutritional supplements and moderate lifestyle changes.

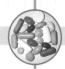

SUPPLEMENTS

- Calcium: 500–1,000 mg daily (older women: 1,500–2,000 mg).
- Coenzyme Q_{10}: 60 mg, one to three times daily.
- Glutathione: 50 mg, one to three times daily.
- Inositol hexanicotinate (no-flush niacin): 250–500 mg daily.
- L-Carnitine: 50–500 mg daily.
- Magnesium: 250–500 mg daily.
- Policosanal: 10 mg daily.
- Vitamin A: 5,000–10,000 IU daily.
- Vitamin C: 500–1,000 mg daily.
- Vitamin D: 200–800 IU daily.
- Vitamin E: 400–500 IU daily.
- Vitamin K: 100 mcg daily.

HERBS

- Cayenne: as directed on label.
- Garlic: 500 mg daily.
- Green tea extract: 100 mg, twice daily.

TRY

- Eat fish, berries, olive oil, fiber-rich foods, whole grains, soy products, and yogurt.
- Exercise regularly.
- Lose weight if necessary.

AVOID / WATCH OUT FOR

- Cholesterol-lowering drugs.
- Fried foods.
- Rancid fats and hydrogenated oils.

Chronic Fatigue Syndrome (CFS)

Chronic fatigue syndrome (CFS) is a disorder characterized by extreme fatigue, low-grade fever, headaches, muscle aches, and impaired memory and/or concentration. The cause of this condition, which can last from twenty-four hours to several years, remains unknown. Care should be taken to rule out other causes of fatigue as a number of conditions may cause similar symptoms. If CFS is the problem, natural remedies can increase energy and relieve the associated aches and pains. See also FATIGUE.

CHRONIC FATIGUE SYNDROME (CFS)

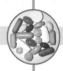

SUPPLEMENTS

- Coenzyme Q_{10}: 60 mg, one to three times daily.
- DHEA: 25 mg daily for women over forty; 50 mg daily for men over forty.
- L-Carnitine: 50–500 mg daily.
- Kelp: 150 mcg daily.
- Vitamin B complex: 25–50 mg daily.
- Zinc: 15 mg of elemental zinc (read label), once or twice daily.

HERBS

- Siberian ginseng: as directed on label.
- Suma: as directed on label.

TRY

- Eat grains, poultry, fish, eggs, beans, nuts, soy products, vegetables, and fruit.
- Yoga and deep breathing exercises.

AVOID / WATCH OUT FOR

- Coffee.
- Refined carbohydrates.
- Sugar.

Circulation, Poor

Poor circulation can affect any area of the body,
but people with this condition commonly
complain of having cold or numb hands and/or
feet. Poor circulation can be a symptom of an
underlying medical condition, which should be
ruled out, or it may simply be the body's
reaction to extreme changes in temperature.
In either case, there are several natural ways
to improve the body's circulation to reduce
the discomfort associated with this condition.

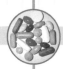

SUPPLEMENTS

- Calcium: 500–1,000 mg daily (older women: 1,500–2,000 mg).
- Coenzyme Q_{10}: 60 mg, one to three times daily.
- L-Carnitine: 50–500 mg daily.
- Magnesium: 250–500 mg daily.
- Omega-3 fatty acids (fish oil capsules): 50 mg, one to three times daily.
- Vitamin B complex: 25–50 mg daily.
- Vitamin C: 500–1,000 mg daily.
- Vitamin E: 400–500 IU daily.

HERBS

- Cayenne: as directed on label.
- Ginger extract (EV EXT 77): one to two 170-mg capsules daily.
- Ginkgo biloba extract: 60 mg, one to three times daily.
- Green tea extract: 100 mg, twice daily.
- Hawthorn: as directed on label.

TRY

- Drink red wine.
- Eat more fiber-rich foods.
- Eat more onions.
- Exercise regularly.
- Lose weight if necessary.
- Massage.

AVOID / WATCH OUT FOR

- Hydrogenated oils.
- Processed foods.
- Smoking.
- Sugar.

Colds and Flu

The common cold and the flu, or influenza, are both caused by a variety of viruses, and both are highly contagious. Symptoms of a cold include sneezing, runny nose, and watery eyes, usually without a fever. The flu, on the other hand, has several additional symptoms, including chills, fever, and sometimes nausea and vomiting. Both conditions respond well to natural remedies. In fact, during cold and flu season, natural remedies can help boost your resistance to these viruses.

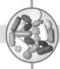

SUPPLEMENTS

- Selenium: 100–200 mcg daily.
- Vitamin A: 5,000–10,000 IU daily.
- Vitamin C: 500–1,000 mg daily.
- Vitamin E: 400–500 IU daily.
- Zinc lozenges: one lozenge dissolved in mouth, two to three times daily.

HERBS

- Echinacea: as directed on label.
- Elderberry: as directed on label.
- Feverfew: as directed on label.
- Garlic: 500 mg daily.
- Ginger extract (EV EXT 77): one to two 170-mg capsules daily.
- Goldenseal: as directed on label.
- Slippery elm: as directed on label.

TRY

- Drink hot liquids (chicken soup and teas).
- Drink more fluids.
- Facial steam with a few drops of eucalyptus oil.
- Get extra rest.
- Saltwater nasal drops.

AVOID / WATCH OUT FOR

- Overdoing it.
- Stress.
- Sugar.

Colon Cancer

Colon cancer is cancer of the large intestines. Diet, heredity, ulcerative colitis, and Crohn's disease all seem to play a part in increasing the risk of developing this disease. Once discovered, the infected segment of the intestines is usually surgically removed. Certain dietary changes, as well as taking nutritional supplements, may decrease the likelihood of cancer developing elsewhere in the intestines. See also CANCER PREVENTION; RECTAL CANCER.

SUPPLEMENTS

- Calcium: 500–1,000 mg daily (older women: 1,500–2,000 mg).
- Folic acid: 400–800 mg daily.

HERBS

- Psyllium: as directed on label.

TRY

- Eat more fresh fruits and vegetables.
- Eat oat fiber.
- Eat soy foods, including soy shakes.

AVOID / WATCH OUT FOR

- High-fat foods.
- Low-fiber foods.

Constipation

Constipation—uncomfortable, infrequent bowel movements—can be either an acute or a chronic condition. The causes of acute constipation can include taking prescription drugs, recent inactivity, or a change in dietary habits. Chronic constipation can be caused by any number of conditions, but is most often due to a lack of dietary fiber. Constipation responds well to nutritional supplements and moderate lifestyle changes. See also DIGESTIVE DISORDERS.

SUPPLEMENTS

- Magnesium: 250–500 mg daily.
- Probiotics: one to three capsules or one tablespoon of refrigerated liquid probiotics, up to three times daily before meals; or acidophilus: one to three (multi-billion count) capsules before meals.
- Vitamin C: 500–1,000 mg daily.

HERBS

- Aloe vera juice: one tablespoon twice daily.
- Cascara sagrada: as directed on label.
- Flaxseed oil (refrigerated): 1 tsp of the oil; or one to three 500 mg capsules daily.
- Psyllium: as directed on label.
- Senna: as directed on label.

TRY

- Detoxification (see TOXICITY on page 186).
- Drink six to eight glasses of pure water daily.
- Eat more fresh vegetables and fruits.
- Eat prunes and bran.
- Exercise regularly.

AVOID / WATCH OUT FOR

- Extended travel.
- Iron supplements.
- Prescription drugs.
- Sugar, cheese, and refined white flour.

Cough

Coughing is an attempt by the body to protect the lungs. Coughs can have many causes, ranging from allergies, respiratory infection, and bronchitis to lung cancer, pneumonia, and tuberculosis. Simple coughing, associated with the common cold for example, can be soothed naturally without the need for commonly used over-the-counter cough medicines.

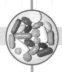

SUPPLEMENTS

- Magnesium: 250–500 mg daily.
- NAC (N-acetylcysteine): 1,500 mg with meals (for bronchitis).
- Vitamin A: 5,000–10,000 IU daily.
- Vitamin C: 500–1,000 mg daily.
- Vitamin E: 400–500 IU daily.

HERBS

- Chickweed: as directed on the label.
- Ginger root tea: drink daily.
- Licorice root: one to three 450-mg capsules daily.
- Mullein: as directed on label.

TRY

- Clean the ventilation system in your home and office.
- Homeopathic cough remedy.
- Humidifier.

AVOID / WATCH OUT FOR

- Candidiasis.
- Cigarette smoke.
- Dust.
- Excess sugar consumption.

Cystitis

A bladder infection (cystitis) is a lower urinary tract infection caused by bacteria. Bladder infections are more common in women than in men. Symptoms include an urgent, frequent desire to urinate and pain during urination. There may also be lower back pain and pain above the pubic bone. Antibiotics are often prescribed for bladder infections; however, this infection responds very well to natural remedies. See also URINARY TRACT INFECTION.

SUPPLEMENTS

- Multivitamin/mineral/antioxidant formula: as directed on label.

HERBS

- Acidophilus: one to three (multi-billion count) capsules before each meal.
- Alfalfa: as directed on label.
- Barberry: as directed on label.
- Cinnamon: as directed on label.
- Cranberry extract capsules: as directed on label.
- Garlic: 500 mg daily.
- Uva ursi: as directed on label.

TRY

- Drink six to ten glasses of pure water daily.
- Drink two 8-ounce glasses of unsweetened cranberry juice daily.
- Wear cotton undergarments.

AVOID / WATCH OUT FOR

- Beans.
- Chocolate.
- Feminine hygiene sprays.
- Refined carbohydrates and sugar.
- Talcum powder.

Dandruff

Dandruff, those annoying flakes of skin that fall from the scalp, is actually part of a skin condition known as seborrheic dermatitis. The face and occasionally other areas of the body can also be affected. While topical medications and prescription shampoos are often prescribed for this condition, dandruff can easily be remedied naturally. Quite often, simple dietary changes and nutritional supplementation are all that's required.

SUPPLEMENTS

- Biotin: 300 mcg daily.
- Folic acid: 400–800 mg daily.
- Kelp: 150 mcg daily.
- Selenium: 100–200 mcg daily.
- Vitamin B_6 (pyridoxine): 25–50 mg daily.
- Vitamin B_{12}: 100–1,000 mcg daily.
- Vitamin E: 400–500 IU daily.
- Zinc: 15 mg of elemental zinc (read label), once or twice daily.

HERBS

- Dandelion: as directed on label.
- Flaxseed oil (refrigerated): 1 tsp of the oil; or one to three 500 mg capsules daily.
- Goldenseal: as directed on label.

TRY

- Eat more fish.
- Eat more raw fruits and vegetables.
- Eat yogurt with live cultures.

AVOID / WATCH OUT FOR

- Dairy products.
- Greasy lotions.
- Irritating shampoo or soaps.
- Nuts, sugar, and fried foods.

Depression

Depression is not merely the blues. It's a serious mood disorder that can have many contributing causes, which aren't fully understood. While it's normal to feel sad occasionally, depression is a lingering, intense sadness that can persist for months or years. Antidepressant drugs are commonly prescribed for depression but carry with them many side effects. Natural remedies can help improve mood and eventually restore a balanced feeling of well-being.

SUPPLEMENTS

- DHEA: 25 mg daily for women over forty;
  50 mg daily for men over forty.
- Magnesium: 250–500 mg daily.
- Pregnenolone: 10 mg daily.
- Vitamin B complex: 25–50 mg daily.

HERBS

- Kava: as directed on label.
- Licorice root: one to three 450-mg capsules daily.
- St. John's wort/phenol complex: 300 mg,
  once or twice daily.

TRY

- Detoxification (see TOXICITY on page 186).
- Exercise regularly.
- Get sufficient sleep.
- Participate in a sport.

AVOID / WATCH OUT FOR

- Antidepressant drugs and other prescription drugs.
- "Diet" products and extreme dieting.
- Processed foods.
- Too little dietary fat.

Diabetes

Diabetes mellitus is a condition in which the body either doesn't produce enough insulin to keep blood sugar at normal levels (type 1, or insulin-dependent diabetes), or the cells do not properly respond to the insulin (type 2, or non–insulin-dependent diabetes). While diabetes is a serious condition that has many long-term complications, it is possible to take natural steps under a doctor's supervision to stabilize blood sugar levels and improve the overall condition.

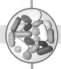

SUPPLEMENTS

- Alpha lipoic acid: 50 mg daily.
- Chromium: 200–600 mg daily.
- Magnesium: 250–500 mg daily.
- MSM: 1,000 mg, one to three times daily.
- Vanadium (Vanadyl): 10 mg daily.
- Vitamin B_6 (pyridoxine): 25–50 mg daily.
- Vitamin E: 400–500 IU daily.

HERBS

- Banaba leaf extract: 60 mg at the end of each meal.
- Bilberry extract: as directed on label.
- Garlic: 500 mg daily.
- Ginkgo biloba extract: 60 mg, one to three times daily.

TRY

- Drink six to ten glasses of pure water daily.
- Increase fiber.
- Lose weight if necessary.
- Reduce carbohydrates.

AVOID / WATCH OUT FOR

- Alcohol.
- Low-fiber foods.
- Refined carbohydrates.
- Saturated fats.
- Soft drinks.
- Sugary desserts.

Diarrhea

Frequent watery bowel movements accompanied by powerful cramping, commonly known as diarrhea, can be a symptom of many different conditions, including gastroenteritis, irritable bowel syndrome, ulcerative colitis, infection with the salmonella bacteria, and so on. Diarrhea that persists for more than a few days or recurs often should be brought to a doctor's attention; however, occasional bouts with diarrhea can be treated naturally and quite easily at home. See also DIGESTIVE DISORDERS.

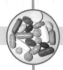

SUPPLEMENTS

- Acidophilus: one to three (multi-billion count) capsules before each meal.
- Calcium: 500–1,000 mg daily (older women: 1,500–2,000 mg).
- Digestive enzymes: one to three capsules with each meal.
- Kelp: 150 mcg daily.
- Potassium: 99 mg, one to three times daily.

HERBS

- Chamomile tea: drink three times daily.
- Garlic: 500 mg daily.
- Raspberry leaves tea: drink three times daily.

TRY

- Drink pure water in excess of six to eight glasses daily.
- Eat fresh fruit and vegetables, including carrots.
- Eat more fiber.
- Eat more whole grains.
- Eat yogurt with live cultures.

AVOID / WATCH OUT FOR

- Dairy products.
- Excess magnesium.

Digestive Disorders

The mouth, throat, esophagus, stomach, small and large intestines, rectum, and anus comprise the digestive tract. Some organs outside the digestive tract—the liver, gallbladder, and pancreas—are actually part of the digestive system. Digestive disorders include any malfunction in any part of the digestive system; however, gastritis, a disorder of the stomach, is a common complaint. This condition, of which there are several causes, can quite often be relieved by taking certain supplements and drinking plenty of water. See also CONSTIPATION; DIARRHEA; ULCER, PEPTIC.

SUPPLEMENTS

- Acidophilus: one to three (multi-billion count) capsules before each meal.
- Digestive enzymes: one to three capsules with each meal.
- MSM: 1,000 mg, one to three times daily.
- Potassium: 99 mg, one to three times daily.

HERBS

- No herbs apply.

TRY

- Drink six to eight glasses of pure water daily.

Ear Infection

Pain in the ear can be caused by any number of factors, including bacteria, injury, fluid buildup, and accumulated pus. The outer ear, middle ear, or inner ear may be affected. Ear infections that are caused by bacteria, such as "swimmer's ear," are commonly treated with antibiotics. Nutritional and herbal supplements, however, are very effective at clearing up ear infections without any of the side effects associated with antibiotics.

SUPPLEMENTS

- Acidophilus: one to three (multi-billion count) capsules before each meal.
- Multivitamin/mineral/antioxidant formula: as directed on label.

HERBS

- Echinacea: as directed on label.
- Garlic: 500 mg daily.

TRY

- Eat soy products.
- Liquid garlic, warmed and dropped into ear canal; plug with cotton for 10 to 15 minutes.

AVOID / WATCH OUT FOR

- Dairy products.
- Excessive use of antibiotics.

Emotional/Physical Lows

It's perfectly normal to sometimes feel sad, tired, agitated, anxious, and so on. And it isn't always obvious why you're feeling that way. While there are a number of prescription drugs to counteract your negative feelings—whether they are physical or emotional—a much better and safer way to improve your condition is to inhale the essences of essential oils. Whatever the desired outcome, within moments of inhalation, you should begin feeling better. See AROMATHERAPY on page 208.

AROMATHERAPY FOR EMOTIONAL/PHYSICAL LOWS

If you're feeling . . .	Try inhaling essence of. . .	For the effect of. . .
Agitated	Bergamot	Restfulness
Anxious	Catnip	Calmness
Forgetful	Lily of the valley	Improved memory
Inner turmoil	Lily	Inner peace
Sad	Apple	Cheerfulness
Unable to sleep	Hops	Sleepiness
Unclean	Hyssop	Purification
Unenergetic	Camphor, ginger, or saffron	Increased energy
Uninterested in sex	Cardamom	Increased sexual desire
Uninterested in sex and loving feelings	Vanilla	Sex and love
Unloved or unloving	Jasmine	Love
Wounded	Eucalyptus or myrrh	Healing

Fatigue

Simple fatigue, as opposed to chronic fatigue, is usually a result of lifestyle factors that stress the body, such as a lack of sufficient sleep, lack of proper nutrition, strenuous physical activity, and smoking. If it is not accompanied by other symptoms that may indicate a more serious problem, fatigue responds quite well to natural remedies, including getting a sufficient amount of sleep nightly. If persistent fatigue is your problem, see CHRONIC FATIGUE SYNDROME.

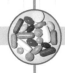

SUPPLEMENTS

- Coenzyme Q_{10}: 60 mg, one to three times daily.
- DHEA: 25 mg daily for women over age 40; 50 mg daily for men over age 40.
- Pregnenolone: 10 mg daily.
- Selenium: 100–200 mcg daily.

HERBS

- Astragalus: as directed on label.
- Buplerum: as directed on label.
- Ginseng: as directed on label.
- Grape seed/green tea complex: 100 mg of each twice daily.

TRY

- Acupuncture.
- Detoxification (see TOXICITY on page 186).
- Exercise regularly.

AVOID / WATCH OUT FOR

- Adrenal exhaustion.
- Candida Infection.
- Environmental toxins.
- Estrogen dominance.
- Food allergens.
- Synthetic hormones (birth control pills and HRT).

Fibromyalgia

Fibromyalgia is a syndrome characterized by chronic pain and stiffness in the muscles, tendons, and ligaments, occurring throughout the body, or sometimes in only one specific area or areas. Pressure to certain spots on the body may cause pain. While the cause of fibromyalgia remains unknown, triggers may include stress, lack of sleep, injury, or infection. It's not necessary to turn to prescription medication for relief, as this condition can be treated naturally.

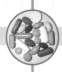

SUPPLEMENTS

- Arginine, time-released: 1,500 mg twice daily.
- Coenzyme Q_{10}: 60 mg, one to three times daily.
- Evening primrose oil capsules: 500–1,000 mg daily.
- Vitamin E: 400–500 IU daily.

HERBS

- Cayenne: as directed on label.
- Grape seed/green tea complex: 100 mg of each twice daily.

TRY

- Acupressure.
- Biofeedback.
- Massage.
- Yoga.

AVOID / WATCH OUT FOR

- Alcohol.
- Caffeine.
- Excess sugar and salt.
- Stress.
- Tobacco.

Fungal Skin Infections

Fungi—of which there are various types in the plant kingdom—are prevalent in our environment. Certain types of fungi can infect the topmost layer (or dead layer) of the skin, causing conditions such as ringworm. Symptoms can range from redness and mild scaling and itching to extremely irritated, blistered skin. Although fungi are difficult to eradicate, natural remedies work well when used for three to six months. See also ATHLETE'S FOOT; CANDIDIASIS.

FUNGAL SKIN INFECTIONS

SUPPLEMENTS

- Acidophilus: one to three (multi-billion count) capsules before each meal.
- Vitamin B complex: 25–50 mg daily.
- Vitamin C: 500–1,000 mg daily.
- Vitamin E: 400–500 IU daily.
- Zinc: 15 mg of elemental zinc (read label), once or twice daily.

HERBS

- Garlic: 500 mg daily.
- Grapefruit seed extract: as directed on label.
- Tea tree oil: apply topically as directed on label.

TRY

- Eat more raw fruits and vegetables.
- Keep infected areas dry.

AVOID / WATCH OUT FOR

- Reduce consumption of meat, grains, and dairy.

Gallstones

Gallstones are crystallized masses of mostly cholesterol that develop in the gallbladder. However, they can also travel to, or occur in, the bile ducts. As long as the stones remain in the gallbladder, this condition can remain silent for many years, or pain of various degrees may come and go. If a gallstone completely obstructs a duct, serious complications can occur. If you're prone to gallstones, there are many natural ways you can reduce the risk of further development.

92   DR. EARL MINDELL'S NATURAL REMEDIES FOR 101 AILMENTS

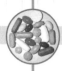

SUPPLEMENTS

- Lecithin granules: one tablespoon, one to three times daily.
- Taurine: 500–1,500 mg daily.

HERBS

- Dandelion: as directed on label.
- Milk thistle (silymarin) capsules: 140 mg, one to three times daily.
- Peppermint: as directed on label.
- Turmeric: as directed on label.

TRY

- Eat oat bran.
- Vegetarian diet.

AVOID / WATCH OUT FOR

- Low-fiber foods.
- Refined carbohydrates.
- Saturated fats.

Gingivitis

Inflammation of the gums is known as gingivitis. The main cause of this condition is plaque buildup along the gum line. Symptoms include red, swollen gums that bleed easily. While brushing and flossing regularly can prevent gum disease, other natural steps—such as including nutritional supplements in your daily regimen—can be taken to improve the condition of your gums.

SUPPLEMENTS

- Beta-carotene: 10,000–20,000 IU daily.
- Coenzyme Q_{10}: 60 mg, one to three times daily.
- Copper: 2–3 mg daily.
- Folic acid: 400–800 mg daily.
- Selenium: 100–200 mcg daily.
- Vitamin C: 500–1,000 mg daily.
- Vitamin E: 400–500 IU daily.
- Zinc: 15 mg of elemental zinc (read label), once or twice daily.

HERBS

- Hawthorn berries: as directed on label.
- Quercetin: 400 mg before eating, one to three times daily.
- Tea tree oil toothpaste: brush regularly.

TRY

- Brush and floss regularly.
- Eat foods high in fiber.
- Eat raw, crunchy vegetables.
- Rinse mouth with mixture of hydrogen peroxide and water.
- Use toothpicks.
- Water irrigation/stimulation.

AVOID / WATCH OUT FOR

- All simple sugars.
- Excess alcohol.
- Refined carbohydrates.
- Smoking.

Gout

Gout is a painful condition in which excess uric acid crystallizes in a joint or joints and causes inflammation (arthritis). Joints commonly affected include those in the feet, knees, wrists, and elbows. Dietary factors, such as high-protein consumption, may play a role in the development of this condition. Natural remedies are aimed at ridding the body of excess uric acid and reducing inflammation.

SUPPLEMENTS

- MSM: 1,000 mg, one to three times daily.
- Multiple antioxidant formula: as directed on label.
- Vitamin B complex: 25–50 mg daily.
- Vitamin B$_6$ (pyridoxine): 25–50 mg daily.

HERBS

- Celery juice: drink daily.
- Cherry juice: drink daily.
- Ginger extract (EV EXT 77): one to two 170-mg capsules daily.
- Grape seed extract (PCOs): 100 mg, one to three times daily.

TRY

- Drink six to eight glasses of pure water daily.
- Reduce protein intake.

AVOID / WATCH OUT FOR

- Excess protein.
- High-purine food, such as organ meats, scallops, mussels, sardines, and herring.

Hair, Skin, and Nail Problems

Hair, skin, and nail problems often occur simultaneously. For example, hair and nails may become dry and brittle, while at the same time the skin becomes dry and flaky. Or hair and skin may become oily, while the nails become soft. Whatever the symptoms, inadequate nutrition is often the culprit in these conditions. It's easy to remedy these problems naturally so that hair regains its glossiness, skin its suppleness, and nails their hardness.

HAIR, SKIN, AND NAILS PROBLEMS

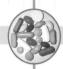

SUPPLEMENTS

- Biotin: 300 mcg daily.
- Calcium: 500–1,000 mg daily (older women: 1,500–2,000 mg).
- Kelp: 150 mcg daily.
- L-Cysteine: 100–250 mg, one to two times daily.
- Magnesium: 250–500 mg daily.
- Selenium: 100–200 mcg daily.
- Vitamin C: 500–1,000 mg daily.
- Vitamin E: 400–500 IU daily.
- Zinc: 15 mg of elemental zinc (read label), once or twice daily.

HERBS

- Aloe vera gel: apply topically as directed on label.
- Dandelion: as directed on label.
- Evening Primrose oil: 500 mg, one to three times daily.
- Horsetail: as directed on the label.
- Oregon grape root: as directed on label.
- Yellow dock: as directed on label.

TRY

- Apply alpha-hydroxy acid to skin as directed on product label.
- Drink six to eight glasses of pure water daily.
- Eat foods high in protein.
- Rinse hair with apple cider or sage tea.
- Wear gloves to protect hands and nails.

AVOID / WATCH OUT FOR

- Excess sun exposure leading to sunburn and/or tanning.
- Excess vitamin A.

Hay Fever

People who suffer from hay fever are allergic to plant pollen. Since trees, grasses, and other plants produce pollen seasonally, hay fever is often referred to as seasonal allergies. Symptoms include sneezing, itchy and watery eyes, and a runny or stuffed nose. When allergy season comes around, many people turn to the widely available prescription and over-the-counter antihistamines, or allergy medicines. What they don't realize is that hay fever can be controlled quite well with natural, time-tested remedies. See also ALLERGIES TO DUST, MOLD, AND DANDER.

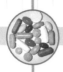

SUPPLEMENTS

- Digestive enzymes: one to three capsules with each meal.
- Magnesium: 250–500 mg daily.
- Vitamin B complex: 25–50 mg daily.
- Vitamin C: 500–1,000 mg daily.
- Zinc: 15 mg of elemental zinc (read label), once or twice daily.

HERBS

- Borage oil: 500–1,000 mg daily (as capsules) *or* evening primrose oil: 500–1,000 mg daily (as capsules).
- Echinacea: as directed on label.
- Ginkgo biloba extract: 60 mg, one to three times daily.
- Grape seed extract (PCOs): 100 mg, one to three times daily.
- Licorice root: one to three 450-mg capsules daily.
- Quercetin: 400 mg before eating, one to three times daily.

TRY

- Colon-cleansing program.
- Detoxification (see TOXICITY on page 186).
- Drink pure water in excess of six to eight glasses daily.
- Immune-system boosters (see IMMUNE SYSTEM, WEAKENED on page 114).

AVOID / WATCH OUT FOR

- Pollen.

Headaches

Some people get headaches frequently, others get them rarely, but virtually everyone has experienced the characteristic throbbing sensation. The causes of headaches vary, and constant recurrence may indicate an underlying condition. However, headaches often have relatively minor causes, such as tension. Relief of a headache can come quite quickly—without the use of aspirin, ibuprofen, acetaminophen, and so on. Common herbs and other natural steps not only bring relief of the actual headache but also may reduce their frequency. See also MIGRAINES.

SUPPLEMENTS

- Calcium: 500–1,000 mg daily (older women: 1,500–2,000 mg).
- DLPA (dl-phenylalanine): 375 mg, one or two capsules every four hours for discomfort.
- Magnesium: 250–500 mg daily.
- Niacin (vitamin B_3): 50–1,000 mg daily, in divided doses.
- Pantothenic acid (vitamin B_5): 30–100 mg daily.
- Vitamin C: 500–1,000 mg daily.
- Vitamin E: 400–500 IU daily.

HERBS

- Chamomile tea: drink one cup daily.
- Feverfew: as directed on label.
- Ginkgo biloba extract: 60 mg, one to three times daily.
- Thyme tea: drink one cup daily.
- White willow bark: one to two 500-mg capsules, two to three times daily.

TRY

- Acupuncture or acupressure.
- Cold compress made with basil tea and witch hazel, applied to forehead.
- Drink six to eight glasses of pure water daily.
- Exercise moderately.
- Massage.

AVOID / WATCH OUT FOR

- Food additives, such as MSG.
- Food allergies.
- Pollen, dust, and environmental toxins.
- Red meat, nuts, chocolate, coffee, and wine.

Hearing Loss

Hearing loss—a deterioration in hearing (as opposed to deafness, which is defined as profound hearing loss)—can have a number of different causes, such as exposure to very loud noise, taking certain drugs, Ménière's disease, stroke, and some hereditary diseases. A buildup of earwax or fluid can also be the culprit. While hearing loss is often irreversible, further deterioration can be avoided by taking protective nutritional supplements and by following some commonsense advice.

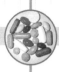

SUPPLEMENTS

- Magnesium: 250–500 mg daily.
- Niacin (vitamin B$_3$): 50–1,000 mg daily, in divided doses.
- Vitamin B$_{12}$: 100–1,000 mcg daily.

HERBS

- Ginkgo biloba extract: 60 mg, one to three times daily.

TRY

- Wear protective headphones/earplugs.

AVOID / WATCH OUT FOR

- Loud noises and music.

Heartburn

Virtually everyone has experienced the pain of heartburn at least once in his or her life, often as a result of eating too much or too fast. Defined as a burning pain behind the breastbone, heartburn is caused by acid reflux, the backflow of stomach contents upward into the esophagus. The pain, which rises in the chest, may extend into the neck, throat, or even face. If you're a frequent sufferer of heartburn, there are a number of natural remedies that you can use to help prevent further occurrences.

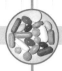

SUPPLEMENTS

- Acidophilus: one to three (multi-billion count) capsules before each meal.
- Betaine hydrochloride (HCL): one 150-mg capsule with each meal.
- Digestive enzymes: one to three capsules with each meal.
- Vitamin B_{12}: 100–1,000 mcg daily.

HERBS

- Aloe vera juice: one tablespoon twice daily.
- Papaya tablets (chewable): one to three tablets after a meal or eat the fruit after a large meal.
- Slippery elm: as directed on label.

TRY

- After eating, stay upright; take a walk.
- Drink a glass of room-temperature water before meals.
- Eat smaller meals slowly.
- Lose excess weight.

AVOID / WATCH OUT FOR

- Antacids.
- Foods and beverages known to trigger heartburn.
- Prescription H2 Blockers, such as Zantac.
- Smoking.

Hemorrhoids

Hemorrhoids are inflamed veins in the wall of the rectum or anus. They can sometimes be painful and occasionally may bleed. Straining during bowel movements is the main cause of this condition. Natural remedies are aimed at relieving pain and reducing inflammation as well as improving the ease of bowel movements.

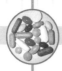

SUPPLEMENTS

- Acidophilus: one to three (multi-billion count) capsules before each meal.
- Rutin: 50 mg, one to three times daily.
- Vitamin C: 500–1,000 mg daily with 500 mg of bioflavonoids daily.
- Vitamin E oil or cream: apply to hemorrhoid.

HERBS

- No herbs apply.

TRY

- Drink six to ten glasses of pure water daily.
- Eat unprocessed bran.
- Exercise regularly.

AVOID / WATCH OUT FOR

- Coffee, chocolate, cola, and cocoa.

Herpes

There are two types of the herpes simplex virus—type I and type II. Type I is the cause of cold sores that form on or around the lips, while type II is the cause of genital herpes. The characteristic blisters are contagious, and care should be taken to avoid skin-to-skin contact. Between outbreaks, the virus lies dormant in the body. Flare-ups often occur during times of stress. Natural remedies can speed the healing of blisters and reduce the frequency of outbreaks.

SUPPLEMENTS

- Lysine: 500 mg before eating, once daily;
  therapeutically 3–4 grams (during a breakout).
- Vitamin A: 5,000–10,000 IU daily.
- Vitamin C: 500–1,000 mg daily with 500 mg
  of bioflavonoids daily.
- Zinc: 15 mg of elemental zinc (read label),
  once or twice daily.

HERBS

- Arnica homeopathic tablets: dissolve under
  tongue as directed on label.
- Calendula ointment or gel: apply topically
  as directed on label.
- Elderberry: as directed on label.
- Licorice root: one to three 450-mg
  capsules daily.

TRY

- Topical witch hazel.

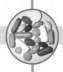

AVOID / WATCH OUT FOR

- Chocolate.
- Coffee.
- Nuts.
- Stress.
- Toothpaste with sodium lauryl sulfate (detergent)
  or sodium laureth sulfate.

Hypoglycemia

Hypoglycemia is a condition in which blood-sugar levels are abnormally low. It is most often found in people with diabetes, as it is a side effect of the diabetic drug insulin. Prolonged fasting or excessive alcohol consumption can, on occasion, also lead to hypoglycemia. Common symptoms of hypoglycemia include sweating, nervousness, faintness, quivering, and, in more serious cases, fatigue, blurry vision, and headaches. Fortunately, many of these symptoms can often be relieved naturally.

HYPOGLYCEMIA

SUPPLEMENTS

- Alpha lipoic acid: 50 mg daily.
- Chromium: 200–600 mg daily.
- Essential fatty acids capsules: 250 mg, one to three times daily.
- Inositol hexanicotinate (no-flush niacin): 250–500 mg daily.
- MSM: 1,000 mg, one to three times daily.
- Vanadium (Vanadyl): 10 mg daily.
- Vitamin C: 500–1,000 mg daily.
- Vitamin E: 400–500 IU daily.

HERBS

- Banaba leaf extract: 60 mg at the end of each meal.
- Ginkgo biloba extract: 60 mg, one to three times daily.
- Ginseng: as directed on label.
- Grape seed extract (PCOs): 100 mg, one to three times daily.

TRY

- Eat more vegetables.
- Exercise regularly.
- Lose weight if necessary.

AVOID / WATCH OUT FOR

- All sugars and refined carbohydrates.
- Excess carbohydrates.
- Processed foods.

Immune System, Weakened

Your immune system is your body's first line of defense against invaders. When your immune system is not functioning at its peak, you are more prone to infection. Many factors, including stress, contribute to a weakened immune system. Also, when your body is busy fighting off one infection, your immune system may not be strong enough to fight another infection developing elsewhere. So, it's always a good idea to help your immune system along by supplementing a healthy diet with immune boosters, such as vitamins and other natural substances.

SUPPLEMENTS

- Beta-carotene: 10,000–20,000 IU daily.
- DHEA: 25 mg daily for women over forty; 50 mg daily for men over forty.
- Glutathione: 50 mg, one to three times daily.
- Melatonin: one to three 1-mg timed-release tablets before bedtime.
- Selenium: 100–200 mcg daily.
- Vitamin B$_6$ (pyridoxine): 25–50 mg daily.
- Vitamin C: 500–1,000 mg daily.
- Zinc: 15 mg of elemental zinc (read label), once or twice daily.

HERBS

- Astragalus: as directed on label.
- Barberry: as directed on label.
- Echinacea: as directed on label.
- Garlic: 500 mg daily.
- Goldenseal: as directed on label.
- Grape seed/green tea complex: 100 mg of each twice daily.
- Oregon grape root: as directed on label.
- Osha: as directed on label.

TRY

- Biofeedback.
- Eat vegetables.
- Eat whole foods.
- Eat yogurt with live cultures.
- Exercise regularly.
- Fresh fruit diet.

AVOID / WATCH OUT FOR

- Sugar.
- Stress.

Impotence

Impotence is a condition in which a man cannot get or maintain an erection to carry out intercourse at least half the time sex is attempted. This condition is quite often attributable to underlying physical problems, and can even be a side effect of certain medications. Making some simple lifestyle changes as well as supplementing the diet with nutrients and herbs can go a long way toward remedying this problem.

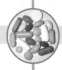

SUPPLEMENTS

- Arginine (timed-release): 1,500 mg, twice daily.
- DHEA: 50 mg daily for men over forty.
- Magnesium: 250–500 mg daily.
- Selenium: 100–200 mcg daily.
- Vitamin A: 5,000–10,000 IU daily.
- Vitamin B complex: 25–50 mg daily.
- Vitamin C: 500–1,000 mg daily.
- Vitamin E: 400–500 IU daily.
- Zinc: 15 mg of elemental zinc (read label), once or twice daily.

HERBS

- Ashwagandha: as directed on label.
- Astragalus: as directed on label.
- Avena sativa: as directed on label.
- Ginkgo biloba extract: 60 mg, one to three times daily.
- Ginseng: as directed on label.
- Gotu kola: as directed on label.
- Yohimbe: as directed on label.

TRY

- Cut down on alcohol consumption.
- Cut down on sugar and fat.
- Drink pure water in excess of eight glasses.
- Reduce stress.

AVOID / WATCH OUT FOR

- Hot tubs and saunas.
- Prescription drugs.
- Smoking.
- Too much exercise.

Indigestion

Almost all of us are familiar with the unpleasant sensation of indigestion, often after we've eaten a big meal. Indigestion, or dyspepsia, is defined as a pain or discomfort in the upper abdomen or chest that's often described as having gas, a feeling of fullness, or a burning pain. It is usually a result of something benign, like anxiety, acid reflux, or lactose intolerance, although it can sometimes indicate a more serious stomach problem. The symptoms of indigestion can usually be treated very effectively using a regimen of natural remedies.

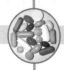

SUPPLEMENTS

- Betaine hydrochloride (HCL): one 150-mg capsule with each meal.
- Digestive enzymes: one to three capsules with each meal.
- Glutamine 50–150 mg daily.
- Probiotics: one to three capsules or one tablespoon of refrigerated liquid probiotics, up to three times daily before meals; or acidophilus: one to three (multi-billion count) capsules before meals.

HERBS

- Cayenne: as directed on label.
- Circumin: as directed on label.
- Fennel: as directed on label.
- Ginger extract (EV EXT 77): one to two 170-mg capsules daily.
- Licorice root: one to three 450-mg capsules daily.
- Mint: as directed on label.

TRY

- Acupuncture.
- Detoxification (see TOXICITY on page 186).
- Eat fiber-rich foods.
- Homeopathic remedy for indigestion.

AVOID / WATCH OUT FOR

- Antacids.
- Antibiotics.
- Fried and fatty foods.
- Heavy metals.
- Prescription H2 Blockers, such as Zantac.
- Refined flours and sugars.

Insomnia

Insomnia is the inability to fall asleep or to stay asleep for a sufficient amount of time during regular sleeping hours. It can last for a few nights or more, or it may occur intermittently. It is often caused by anxiety or depression; it can also be a side effect of certain medications, or drinking caffeinated or alcoholic beverages too close to bedtime. Natural remedies can work quite well to ensure a good night's sleep.

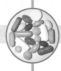

SUPPLEMENTS

- Calcium: 500–1,000 mg daily (older women: 1,500–2,000 mg) before bedtime.
- Inositol: 250–500 mg daily.
- Magnesium: 250–500 mg daily before bedtime.
- Melatonin: one to three 1-mg timed-release tablets before bedtime.
- Vitamin B complex: 25–50 mg daily.

HERBS

- Hops: as directed on label.
- Kava: as directed on label.
- Saw palmetto: as directed on label (for men with prostate problems).
- Skullcap: as directed on label.
- St. John's wort/phenol complex: 300 mg, once or twice daily.
- Valerian: as directed on label.

TRY

- Eat a complex carbohydrate snack a half-hour before bed.
- Exercise regularly.
- Meditation or other stress-relieving techniques.

AVOID / WATCH OUT FOR

- Drugs such as corticosteroids, antidepressants, and cold remedies.
- Excess alcohol, sugar, and caffeine consumption.
- Lots of fluids before bed.
- Muscle tension.

Jet Lag

JET LAG

The cluster of physical and psychological symptoms associated with travel across time zones is known as jet lag. Characterized by fatigue, difficulty sleeping, mental fogginess, and dehydration, jet lag can spoil the first few days of a vacation or business trip. It's best to prepare yourself prior to travel by getting adequate sleep, drinking plenty of fluids, and staying in as good a shape as possible. There are several natural remedies available to help you readjust to the new time zone so that you can enjoy your trip to the fullest.

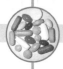

SUPPLEMENTS

- Calcium: 500–1,000 mg daily before bedtime (older women: 1,500–2,000 mg).
- Magnesium: 250–500 mg daily before bedtime.
- Melatonin: one to three 1-mg timed-release tablets before bedtime.
- Vitamin B complex: 25–50 mg daily.
- Vitamin C: 500–1,000 mg daily.

HERBS

- Chamomile: as directed on label.
- Hops: as directed on label.
- Kava: as directed on label.
- Skullcap: as directed on label.
- Valerian: as directed on label.

TRY

- Drink six to ten glasses of pure water daily.
- Homeopathic remedy for jet lag.
- Humidifier.

AVOID / WATCH OUT FOR

- Caffeine.
- Drugs.
- Excess alcohol consumption.
- Excess fluids before bed.
- Gaseous foods while flying.
- Stress.

Kidney Stones

Kidney stones are crystallized stonelike masses of mostly calcium that form in the kidneys. They can range in size from microscopic to an inch or more in diameter. There are many possible causes, including urinary tract infections, heredity, metabolic disorders, and gout. Symptoms may include severe pain, blood in the urine, and a frequent urge to urinate. Drinking plenty of water helps most stones pass out through the urine, and also helps prevent the formation of new ones. There are also a number of other natural steps you can take to remain virtually stone-free.

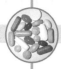

SUPPLEMENTS

- Calcium: 500–1,000 mg daily (older women: 1,500–2,000 mg).
- Magnesium: 250–500 mg daily.
- Potassium: 99 mg, one to three times daily.
- Vitamin B$_6$ (pyridoxine): 25–50 mg daily.

HERBS

- Uva ursi: as directed on label.

TRY

- Drink eight to ten glasses of pure water daily.
- Drink orange juice.
- Eat fresh fruits and vegetables, especially lima beans, apricots, bananas, cantaloupe, and potatoes.
- Eat yogurt with live cultures.

AVOID / WATCH OUT FOR

- Large amounts of oxalate-containing foods, such as animal protein.

Lung Cancer

Lung cancer is the most common cancer in both men and women. The overwhelming majority of lung cancer cases are caused by cigarette smoking. The symptoms of lung cancer vary to some degree, but the main symptom is almost always a persistent cough. The best prevention for lung cancer is to quit smoking, but if you are a longtime smoker, it is highly recommended that you get regular screenings and take nutritional supplements.

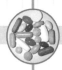

SUPPLEMENTS

- Carotenoids: 10,000–20,000 IU daily.
- Selenium: 100–200 mcg daily.
- Vitamin E: 400–500 IU daily.

HERBS

- Grape seed/green tea complex: 100 mg of each twice daily.

TRY

- Eat raw vegetables and fruits.

AVOID / WATCH OUT FOR

- Automobile fumes.
- Secondhand smoke.
- Smoking.

Macular Degeneration

Macular degeneration is a degenerative eye disorder that results in a gradual loss of vision generally in both eyes. This disorder tends to be hereditary and usually occurs later in life. It doesn't normally cause complete blindness—peripheral vision is usually unaffected. It's not possible to reverse this disorder; however, further degeneration can be slowed with nutritional supplementation.

MACULAR DEGENERATION

SUPPLEMENTS

- Carotenoids: 10,000–20,000 IU daily.
- Lutein: 6–20 mg daily.
- Multivitamin/mineral/antioxidant formula: as directed on label.
- Selenium: 100–200 mcg daily.
- Vitamin C: 500–1,000 mg daily.
- Zinc: 15 mg of elemental zinc (read label), once or twice daily.

HERBS

- Ginkgo biloba extract: 60 mg, one to three times daily.
- Grape seed/green tea complex: 100 mg of each twice daily.

TRY

- Eat more peas, oysters, and lean meats.

AVOID / WATCH OUT FOR

- High-fat foods.
- Low-fiber foods.
- Smoking.
- Sugar.

Macular Degeneration

Memory Loss

Forgetfulness is often attributed to the normal effects of aging; however, there's no reason an otherwise healthy adult can't retain a sharp memory well into old age. While memory loss can be a symptom of Alzheimer's disease, senile dementia, and other neurodegenerative disorders, it can also simply be a result of inadequate nutrition, lack of sleep, a side effect of certain medications, or other easily remedied problems. Restoring and maintaining a good memory is possible by supplementing the diet with natural memory-promoting nutrients and by making simple lifestyle changes.

MEMORY LOSS

SUPPLEMENTS

- Choline: 500–1,000 mg daily.
- DMAE: 75 mg, once or twice daily.
- Folic acid: 400–800 mg daily.
- L-Carnitine: 50–500 mg daily.
- Pantothenic acid (vitamin B_5): 30–100 mg daily.
- Phosphatidyl serine: 15 mg, once or twice daily.
- Pregnenolone: 10 mg daily.
- Vitamin B_1 (thiamin): 50–500 mg daily.
- Vitamin B_{12}: 100–1,000 mcg daily.
- Zinc: 15 mg of elemental zinc (read label),
  once or twice daily.

HERBS

- Bacopa extract: 100 mg daily.
- Club moss (Huperzine A): as directed on label.
- Fo-ti: as directed on label.
- Ginkgo biloba extract: 60 mg, one to three
  times daily.
- Gotu kola: as directed on label.
- Schizandra: as directed on label.
- Siberian ginseng root: as directed on label.
- Vinpocetine: as directed on label.

TRY

- Exercise regularly.
- Get enough sleep (at least seven to eight hours).
- Yoga.

AVOID / WATCH OUT FOR

- Alcohol.
- Drugs that interfere with brain function.
- High blood pressure.
- Poor diet.
- Stress.

Menopausal Symptoms

Menopause is the period in a woman's life when menstruation stops. It doesn't occur overnight, of course; it can take anywhere from one to two years. Problems associated with menopause can include hot flashes, dryness of the vaginal walls, night sweats, irritability, loss of bone calcium, and depression. Fortunately, there are many natural remedies a woman can use to ease the troublesome symptoms of menopause so that she can pass through this stage of her life in relative comfort. See also VAGINAL DRYNESS.

SUPPLEMENTS

- Calcium: 500–1,000 mg daily (older women: 1,500–2,000 mg).
- Magnesium: 250–500 mg daily.
- NAC (N-acetylcysteine): 1,500 mg with meals daily.
- Natural progesterone cream: use as directed on label.
- Soy isoflavonoids: 40–60 mg daily.
- Vitamin B_6 (pyridoxine): 25–50 mg daily.
- Vitamin C: 500–1,000 mg daily.

HERBS

- Anise: as directed on label.
- Dong quai: as directed on label.
- Fennel: as directed on label.
- Ginseng: as directed on label.
- Licorice root: one to three 450-mg capsules daily.
- Red clover: as directed on label.
- Vitex (chasteberry): as directed on label.

TRY

- Eat more fresh fruits and vegetables.
- Eat soy foods.
- Exercise regularly.
- Lose weight if necessary.
- Natural estrogen cream for vaginal dryness.

AVOID / WATCH OUT FOR

- Excess weight.
- Junk food.
- Lack of exercise.
- Stress.
- Synthetic hormones (HRT).

Migraines

Migraines are recurrent painful headaches, sometimes severe, that commonly affect only one side of the head, but sometimes affect both. They are caused by the restriction and dilation of blood vessels in the head. An attack may last several hours or even days. People who get migraines commonly turn to prescription and over-the-counter medications for relief. However, natural remedies can be just as effective, are safer, and can even reduce the frequency of attacks. See also HEADACHES.

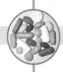

SUPPLEMENTS

- Calcium: 500–1,000 mg daily (older women: 1,500–2,000 mg).
- Magnesium: 250–500 mg daily.
- Niacin (vitamin B$_3$): 50–1,000 mg daily, in divided doses.
- Vitamin B complex: 25–50 mg daily.

HERBS

- Feverfew: as directed on label.
- Ginkgo biloba extract: 60 mg, one to three times daily.
- Peppermint: as directed on label.
- St. John's wort/phenol complex: 300 mg, once or twice daily.
- White willow bark: one to two 500-mg capsules, two to three times daily.

TRY

- Relaxation.
- Use a headband.

AVOID / WATCH OUT FOR

- Alcohol.
- Excess stress.
- Stressor foods, including fat, caffeine, alcohol, sugar, and salt.
- Tobacco.

Muscle Pull

A pulled muscle can be very painful, but the pain is usually not long-lasting. It can occur from overextension or overuse during exercise or even during regular daily activities, such as lifting a child or a heavy household item. To prevent muscle pulls, it is very important to stretch often to maintain muscle flexibility and to warm up properly before workouts. Pushing yourself past your limits should be avoided. Certain steps can help prevent muscle pulls, while others relieve the pain once the pull has occurred. See also SPRAINS AND STRAINS.

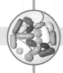

SUPPLEMENTS

- Vitamin B_6 (pyridoxine): 25–50 mg daily.
- Vitamin B_{12}: 100–1,000 mcg daily.
- Vitamin C: 500–1,000 mg daily with 500 mg of bioflavonoids daily.

HERBS

- Arnica ointment: apply topically as directed on label.
- Eucalyptus ointment: apply topically as directed on label.
- Grape seed extract (PCOs): 100 mg, one to three times daily.
- White willow bark: one to two 500-mg capsules, two to three times daily.

TRY

- Drink six ounces of water every fifteen to twenty minutes while exercising.
- Stretch before workouts.

AVOID / WATCH OUT FOR

- Cola drinks.
- Fried foods.
- Refined flour.
- Strenuous exercise.
- White sugar.

Nausea

Nausea is the uncomfortable feeling in the stomach that usually precedes vomiting, but it can also occur alone. There are a number of causes, including motion sickness, certain drugs, flu, and even psychological problems, to name just a few. When a person is nauseous, immediate relief of the unpleasant feeling is highly desired. Vomiting usually brings relief— at least for a little while. Natural remedies work to settle the stomach and bypass the need to vomit.

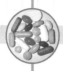

SUPPLEMENTS

- Glutamine: 50–150 mg daily.
- Vitamin B complex: 25–50 mg daily.
- Vitamin B_6 (pyridoxine): 25–50 mg daily.
- Vitamin C: 500–1,000 mg daily.
- Vitamin K: 100 mcg daily.

HERBS

- Basil: as directed on label.
- Chamomile: as directed on label.
- Ginger extract (EV EXT 77): one to two 170-mg capsules daily.
- Kava: as directed on label.
- Licorice root: one to three 450-mg capsules daily.
- Peppermint tea: drink as needed.

TRY

- Acupressure.
- Detoxification (see TOXICITY on page 186).

AVOID / WATCH OUT FOR

- Greasy foods.
- Overeating.
- Prescription drugs.

Oral Cancer

Oral cancer predominantly affects those over the age of forty, although it can affect certain young people who abuse chewing tobacco. The most common cause of oral cancer, like lung cancer, is cigarette smoking. Early signs of the disease include a lump or mass on the inside of the mouth or a white or red patch of tissue in the mouth that refuses to heal. As with lung cancer, the best prevention for oral cancer is to quit smoking.

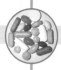

SUPPLEMENTS

- Beta-carotene: 10,000–20,000 IU daily.
- Multiple antioxidant formula: as directed on label.
- Spirulina: 1,000 mg, one to three times daily.
- Vitamin E: 400–500 IU daily.

HERBS

- Green tea extract: 100 mg, twice daily, or drink one cup of tea daily.

TRY

- Eat darkly colored fresh fruits and vegetables.

AVOID / WATCH OUT FOR

- Excessive alcohol consumption.
- Tobacco (all forms).

Osteoporosis

Osteoporosis is a thinning of the bones that can eventually lead to fractures and deformity. It is usually the result of a progressive decrease in calcium reabsorption into the bones and is most common in postmenopausal women and the elderly. Common symptoms of osteoporosis include painful backaches and frequent fractures. Osteoporosis, however, is not a necessary evil of old age. It can often be treated effectively or even be prevented with a complete regimen of natural remedies.

SUPPLEMENTS

- Acidophilus: one to three (multi-billion count) capsules before meals.
- Boron: 2 mg daily.
- Calcium: 500–1,000 mg daily (older women: 1,500–2,000 mg).
- Omega-3 fatty acids (fish oil capsules): 50 mg, one to three times daily.
- Magnesium: 250–500 mg daily.
- Manganese: 9 mg daily.
- Vitamin D: 200–800 IU daily.
- Zinc: 15 mg of elemental zinc (read label), once or twice daily.

HERBS

- Butcher's broom: as directed on label.
- Garlic: 500 mg daily.
- Grape seed extract (PCOs): 100 mg, one to three times daily.
- Horsetail: as directed on label.
- Licorice root: one to three 450-mg capsules daily.

TRY

- Eat soy products.
- Gentle weight-bearing exercises.
- Natural progesterone cream.

AVOID / WATCH OUT FOR

- Excess caffeinated sodas (leaches calcium from bone).
- Excess protein (leaches calcium from bone).
- Prescription drugs, such as cortisones and corticosteroids.

Overweight

Overweight is a condition in which a person has some excess body fat. While it is not as serious as obesity (weighing 20 percent more than the average recommended weight for height and sex), excess body fat stresses the body, contributes to low self-esteem, and can lead to obesity, which carries with it risk of disease. Although losing weight seems like a difficult task, once a person has set his or her mind to following some simple natural guidelines, including regular exercise, healthy weight loss is well within reach.

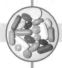

SUPPLEMENTS

- Chromium: 200–600 mg daily.
- Vanadium (Vanadyl): 10 mg daily.

HERBS

- Banaba leaf extract: 60 mg at the end of each meal.
- Gymnema sylvestre: as directed on label.
- Marshmallow extract: as directed on label.

TRY

- Drink six to ten glasses of pure water daily.
- Exercise regularly.
- Reduce carbohydrate intake.

AVOID / WATCH OUT FOR

- Estrogen and synthetic progestins (birth control pills and HRT).
- Lack of exercise.
- Stress.
- Sugary, fatty, and refined foods.

Pain

PAIN

Everyone has experienced some kind of pain
at one time or another. Pain is defined as an
unpleasant sensation signaling that the body
is damaged or threatened by an injury. Pain
can result from a wide range of causes, from
lacerations, fractures, and bruises to diseases
such as cancer, arthritis, and AIDS. Most people
turn to some type of analgesic (pain reliever)
such as aspirin, codeine, or morphine to treat
their pain. However, it can often be treated as
effectively with the use of a variety of natural
methods, which do not have the potentially
serious side effects of drugs.

SUPPLEMENTS

- Choline: 500–1,000 mg daily.
- Digestive enzymes: one to three capsules with each meal.
- DLPA (dl-phenylalanine): 375 mg, one or two capsules every four hours for discomfort.
- Ginger extract (EV EXT 77): one to two 170-mg capsules daily.
- Glucosamine hydrochlorida: 600–1,200 mg daily.
- Vitamin B_1 (thiamin): 50–500 mg daily.
- Vitamin B complex: 25–50 mg daily.

HERBS

- Aloe vera gel (cuts, wounds, and burns): apply topically as directed on label.
- Arnica gel (bruising and swelling): apply topically as directed on label.
- Calendula ointment or gel: apply topically as directed on label.
- Capsaicin: as directed on label.
- Feverfew (headache): as directed on label.
- White willow bark: one to two 500-mg capsules, two to three times daily.

TRY

- Acupuncture/acupressure.
- Alternate between hot and cold packs.
- Exercise regularly.
- Meditation, tai chi, and/or yoga.

AVOID / WATCH OUT FOR

- Coffee.
- Improper lifting (back pain).
- NSAIDs (nonsteroidal anti-inflammatory drugs).
- Stress.

Premenstrual Syndrome (PMS)

PMS is a condition in which a variety of symptoms, including nervousness, irritability, depression, headaches, tissue swelling, and breast tenderness, may occur up to fourteen days before a woman starts her period. It usually disappears soon after the period begins. Although women often turn to over-the-counter drugs for relief, there are a number of natural remedies that can be used to alleviate many of the troublesome symptoms of PMS.

PREMENSTRUAL SYNDROME (PMS)

SUPPLEMENTS

- Calcium: 500–1,000 mg daily (older women: 1,500–2,000 mg).
- Essential fatty acids capsules: 250 mg, one to three times daily.
- Iron (organic): 10–15 mg of essential iron daily
- Magnesium: 250–500 mg daily.
- Manganese: 9 mg daily.
- Multivitamin: as directed on label.
- Soy isoflavonoids: 40–60 mg daily.
- Vitamin A: 5,000–10,000 IU daily.
- Vitamin B_6 (pyridoxine): 25–50 mg daily.
- Vitamin C: 500–1,000 mg daily.
- Vitamin E: 400–500 IU daily.
- Zinc: 15 mg of elemental zinc (read label), once or twice daily.

HERBS

- Dong quai: as directed on label.
- Ginkgo biloba extract: 60 mg, one to three times daily.
- Licorice root: one to three 450-mg capsules daily.
- Milk thistle (silymarin): 140 mg, one to three times daily.
- Vitex (chasteberry): as directed on label.
- Wild yam: as directed on label.

TRY

- Eat dandelion greens and other leafy green vegetables.
- Eat more protein and fewer fats.
- Exercise regularly and do gentle weightlifting.

AVOID / WATCH OUT FOR

- Birth control pills/synthetic hormones.
- Dairy products, refined carbohydrates, and sugar.
- Estrogen dominance.
- Excess colas or other caffeinated soda and coffee.

Prostate, Enlarged

The prostate is a small gland nestled around the urethra, the duct that drains the bladder. In many men over age forty-five, the gland tends to gradually grow larger. If the gland grows too large, it can begin to squeeze the urethra, making urination difficult. Those who suffer from an enlarged prostate often feel the need to urinate more frequently and feel that their urinations are incomplete. Treatment of this condition usually focuses on shrinking the prostate, which can often be accomplished using a variety of natural remedies. See also PROSTATE CANCER.

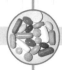

SUPPLEMENTS

- Glycine: 50 mg, one to three times daily.
- Glutamine: 50–150 mg daily.
- Selenium: 100–200 mcg daily.
- Vitamin B$_6$ (pyridoxine): 25–50 mg daily.
- Vitamin C: 500–1,000 mg daily.
- Vitamin E: 400–500 IU daily.
- Zinc: 15 mg of elemental zinc (read label), once or twice daily.

HERBS

- Nettles: as directed on label.
- Pygeum: as directed on label.
- Saw palmetto: as directed on label.

TRY

- Drink six to eight glasses of pure water daily.
- Eat pumpkin seeds, a good source of zinc.
- Eat soy products, cold-water fish, fresh fruits and vegetables, and yogurt with live cultures.

AVOID / WATCH OUT FOR

- Excess alcohol consumption.
- Fatty foods and junk foods.
- Hydrogenated oils.
- Stress.
- Sugar.

Prostate Cancer

Cancer of the prostate is extremely common in elderly men, though its exact cause isn't known. It tends to grow very slowly over a period of many years and eventually gives symptoms similar to those of an enlarged prostate, if any. The best prevention for prostate cancer is early detection, and regular prostate screenings for men over age forty-five are highly recommended. See also PROSTATE, ENLARGED.

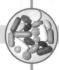

SUPPLEMENTS

- Lutein: 6–20 mg daily.
- Lycopene: 6–10 mg daily.
- Multivitamin/mineral/antioxidant formula: as directed on label.
- Soy isoflavonoids: 40–60 mg daily.

HERBS

- No herbs apply.

TRY

- Eat soybeans and tofu.

AVOID / WATCH OUT FOR

- Diet high in saturated fats.

Psoriasis/Eczema

Psoriasis and eczema are both very common diseases of the skin that are accompanied by scaling, inflammation, itchiness, and redness. Although both are rarely serious, they are often very uncomfortable and can make those who suffer from them self-conscious. With the use of natural methods, however, psoriasis and eczema can often be treated and controlled very effectively.

SUPPLEMENTS

- Omega-3 fatty acids (fish oil capsules): 50 mg, one to three times daily.
- Selenium: 100–200 mcg daily.
- Vitamin A: 5,000–10,000 IU daily.
- Vitamin D: 200–800 IU daily.

HERBS

- Aloe vera gel: apply topically as directed on label.
- Capsaicin: as directed on label.
- Yellow dock: as directed on label.

TRY

- Lose weight if necessary.

AVOID / WATCH OUT FOR

- Excess alcohol consumption.
- High-fat foods.
- Stress.

Rectal Cancer

Rectal cancer is very closely linked to colon cancer, and the diseases together are often referred to as colorectal cancer. Diet and heredity both seem to play major roles in increasing the risk of developing this disease. Common symptoms of rectal cancer include blood in the stool, change in bowel habits, and frequent vomiting. Certain dietary changes, as well as the use of nutritional supplements, may help in the prevention of rectal cancer. See also COLON CANCER.

SUPPLEMENTS

- Calcium: 500–1,000 mg daily (older women: 1,500–2,000 mg).
- Folic acid: 400–800 mg daily.

HERBS

- Psyllium: as directed on label.

TRY

- Eat nuts, fruits, and vegetables.
- Eat oat fiber.
- Eat soy foods, including soy protein shakes.

AVOID / WATCH OUT FOR

- Low-fiber foods.
- Saturated fats.

Restless Leg Syndrome

Also known as Ekbom syndrome, restless leg syndrome is a condition in which an irritating sense of uneasiness and itching, often accompanied by twitching and pain, is felt in the calves of the legs when sitting or lying. The only relief is walking or moving the legs, which unfortunately sometimes leads to insomnia. Natural remedies, however, can often help to alleviate the symptoms of this condition.

RESTLESS LEG SYNDROME

SUPPLEMENTS

- Calcium: 500–1,000 mg daily (older women: 1,500–2,000 mg).
- Vitamin E: 400–500 IU daily.

HERBS

- Butcher's broom: as directed on label.
- Ginkgo biloba extract: 60 mg, one to three times daily.
- Horse chestnut: as directed on label.

TRY

- Exercise regularly.

AVOID / WATCH OUT FOR

- Sitting in one position for a long time.

Senile Dementia

Senile dementia is defined as the loss of intellectual faculties, often associated with behavioral deterioration, beginning for the first time in old age. Most people who suffer from this disease have impaired memory, judgment, and learning ability, and often their personalities deteriorate. The most common causes of senile dementia are Alzheimer's disease and strokes. With the aid of natural therapies, the symptoms of senile dementia can often be alleviated and sometimes even be prevented.

SENILE DEMENTIA

SUPPLEMENTS

- Coenzyme Q$_{10}$: 60 mg, one to three times daily.
- DHEA: 25 mg daily for women over forty;
  50 mg daily for men over forty.
- Folic acid: 400–800 mg daily.
- NADH: 10 mg on an empty stomach daily.
- Natural progesterone cream: use as directed
  on label (for women).
- Niacin: 50–1,000 mg daily, in divided doses.
- Vitamin B$_{12}$: 100–1,000 mcg daily.
- Vitamin C: 500–1,000 mg daily.
- Vitamin E: 400–500 IU daily.
- Zinc: 15 mg of elemental zinc (read label),
  once or twice daily.

HERBS

- Bacopa extract: 100 mg daily.
- Club moss (Huperzine A): as directed on label.
- Ginkgo biloba extract: 60 mg, one to three
  times daily.

TRY

- Drink pure water in excess of eight glasses daily.
- Eat high-fiber foods and more protein.

AVOID / WATCH OUT FOR

- Aluminum foil and cookware.
- Environmental toxins, such as pesticides.
- Fumes from solvents, paints, and glues.
- Prescription drugs.
- Vitamin B$_{12}$ deficiency.

Sinusitis

Inflammation of the sinuses (the hallow cavities in the bones around the nose) is known as sinusitis. It is usually due to allergy or to a bacterial, viral, or fungal infection. It can be either a short-lived or an ongoing condition. Symptoms of sinusitis include pain below the eyes and over the cheeks, headache, and toothache. Antibiotics are often prescribed, and sometimes, over-the-counter remedies are used. However, natural remedies work just as well and do not have the associated side effects of common medications. See also ALLERGIES; HAY FEVER; TOOTHACHE.

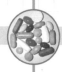

SUPPLEMENTS

- Coenzyme Q_{10}: 60 mg, one to three times daily.
- MSM: 1,000 mg, one to three times daily.
- Vitamin A: 5,000–10,000 IU daily.
- Vitamin B complex: 25–50 mg daily.
- Vitamin C: 500–1,000 mg daily.
- Zinc: 15 mg of elemental zinc (read label), once or twice daily.

HERBS

- Echinacea: as directed on label.
- Garlic: 500 mg daily.
- Goldenseal: as directed on label.

TRY

- Drink hot liquids.
- Drink pure water in excess of eight glasses daily.
- Eat more raw fruits and vegetables.
- Nasal irrigation with water, salt, and baking soda solution.

AVOID / WATCH OUT FOR

- Allergenic foods.
- Dairy products.
- Dust and pollen.
- Forceful nose blowing.
- Irritant fumes and smoke.
- Overuse of decongestants.

Skin Cancer

Skin cancer is the most common type of cancer, but most types are curable. The more common forms of skin cancer usually develop on sun-exposed areas. People who have had a lot of sun exposure, particularly those with fair complexions, are most likely to develop this type of cancer. A telltale sign of skin cancer is the emergence of a new growth or enlarging mole on the surface of the skin, which should be brought to a doctor's attention as soon as possible.

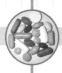

SUPPLEMENTS

- Carotenoids: 10,000–20,000 IU daily.
- Multiple antioxidant formula: as directed on label.
- Vitamin C: 500–1,000 mg daily.

HERBS

- No herbs apply.

TRY

- Eat more vegetables, especially Swiss chard, pumpkin, cabbage, Brussels sprouts, and broccoli.
- Use sun block SPF 15.

AVOID / WATCH OUT FOR

- Diet high in saturated fat.
- Overexposure to sun.

Skin Irritations

There are many different kinds of skin irritations, which can be treated in any number of ways. Acne, rashes, dermatitis, and eczema are all considered irritations of the skin. They are usually marked by a redness or an inflammation on the surface of the skin. Drugstores stock countless products that are aimed at alleviating these irritations, but there are a number of natural therapies that are equally effective in not only treating these irritations, but also preventing further ones from developing.

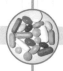

SUPPLEMENTS

- MSM: 1,000 mg, one to three times daily.
- Omega-3 fatty acids (fish oil capsules):
  50 mg, one to three times daily.
- Selenium: 100–200 mcg daily.
- Vitamin A: 5,000–10,000 IU daily.
- Vitamin D: 200–800 IU daily.

HERBS

- Aloe vera gel: apply topically as directed
  on label.
- Capsaicin: as directed on label.
- Gotu kola: as directed on label.

TRY

- Drink six to ten glasses of pure water
  daily.

AVOID / WATCH OUT FOR

- Excessive alcohol consumption.
- High-fat foods.
- Sugar.

Sore Throat

A sore throat is common to anyone who has had a bad cold or flu, or yelled too much at a sporting event. It is defined as a pain at the back of the mouth, which is commonly due to a bacterial or viral infection of the tonsils, larynx, or the pharynx, or to an overuse of the vocal cords. A sore throat can also be an indicator of something more serious, such as a strep throat or mononucleosis. While many people turn to antibiotics, medicated lozenges, and other medicines to treat their sore throats, many natural therapies are just as effective.

SUPPLEMENTS

- Acidophilus: one to three (multi-billion count) capsules before each meal.
- Vitamin A: 5,000–10,000 IU daily.
- Vitamin C: 500–1,000 mg daily.
- Zinc lozenges: one lozenge dissolved in mouth, two to three times daily.

HERBS

- Echinacea: as directed on label.
- Garlic: 500 mg daily.
- Goldenseal: as directed on label.
- Slippery elm: as directed on label.

TRY

- Drink plenty of liquids.
- Gargle with echinacea/goldenseal water or saltwater.
- Swallow 1 tablespoon of honey mixed with lemon juice.

AVOID / WATCH OUT FOR

- Dust and pollen.
- Gum or tooth infections.
- Heavy coughing.
- Smoke and fumes.
- Very hot food and drinks.

Sprains and Strains

Sprains and strains, while often painful, are almost always treatable. A sprain is an injury to a ligament that is usually caused by a sudden overstretching. A strain is the excessive stretching of a muscle, resulting in pain and swelling of the muscle. While the passage of time and reduced use of the affected ligament or muscle is the best remedy, recovery from sprains and strains can be speeded up with the help of a regimen of natural remedies. See also MUSCLE PULL.

SUPPLEMENTS

- Calcium: 500–1,000 mg daily (older women: 1,500–2,000 mg).
- Digestive enzymes: one to three capsules with each meal.
- Magnesium: 250–500 mg daily.
- Vitamin B complex: 25–50 mg daily.
- Vitamin C: 500–1,000 mg daily with 500 mg of bioflavonoids daily.
- Zinc: 15 mg of elemental zinc (read label), once or twice daily.

HERBS

- Aloe vera gel: apply topically as directed on label.
- Arnica gel: apply topically as directed on label.
- Calendula ointment or gel: apply topically as directed on label.

TRY

- Alternate between heat packs and ice packs.
- Eat extra protein.
- Take hot baths with Epsom salts and baking soda.

AVOID / WATCH OUT FOR

- Excess consumption of aspirin, ibuprofen, and acetaminophen.
- Overexercising.

Stomach Cancer

Stomach cancer usually affects older people.
The symptoms of this type of cancer are similar
to those of a peptic ulcer, namely burning,
aching, soreness, and an empty feeling. While
its causes have not been confirmed, dietary
factors are thought to play a key role. Thus,
a healthy diet and a regimen of natural
supplements can be crucial in preventing
this disease.

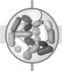

SUPPLEMENTS

- Multiple antioxidant formula: as directed on label.
- Vitamin C: 500–1,000 mg daily.

HERBS

- Garlic: 500 mg daily.
- Grape seed/green tea complex: 100 mg of each twice daily.

TRY

- Eat onions, leeks, chives, garlic, and shallots.

AVOID / WATCH OUT FOR

- Nitrites and nitrates, commonly found in luncheon meats, hot dogs, sausages, jerky, and bacon.

Stress

Stress is any factor that puts a strain on the body. It can be physical or psychological in nature. Stress can result from injury, disease, infection, overwork, financial worries, changes in the environment, relationship conflicts, and even too much of a "good thing." When the body is stressed by any one factor, it is more susceptible to other stressors. When you are stressed-out, try to reduce, treat, or eliminate the stressor from your life, and turn to natural remedies to build up your resistance.

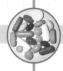

SUPPLEMENTS

- Calcium: 500–1,000 mg daily (older women: 1,500–2,000 mg).
- DHEA: 25 mg daily for women over forty; 50 mg daily for men over forty.
- Magnesium: 250–500 mg daily.
- Melatonin: one to three 1-mg timed-release tablets before bedtime.
- Vitamin B complex: 25–50 mg daily.

HERBS

- Chamomile: as directed on label.
- Kava: as directed on label.
- Siberian ginseng: as directed on label.
- St. John's wort/phenol complex: 300 mg, once or twice daily.
- Valerian: as directed on label.

TRY

- Exercise regularly.
- Massage.

AVOID / WATCH OUT FOR

- Stressor foods, including fat, caffeine, alcohol, sugar, and salt.
- Tobacco.

Stroke

A stroke (apoplexy) is a sudden attack of weakness affecting one side of the body, a consequence of an interruption of the flow of blood to the brain. Early symptoms include slurred speech, becoming dizzy or confused, and blurred or lost vision. Strokes are caused by high blood pressure, diabetes, high cholesterol, and smoking. A program of natural remedies can be very effective in preventing the onset of a stroke, and can also help with recovery. See also CARDIOVASCULAR DISEASE.

SUPPLEMENTS

- Calcium: 500–1,000 mg daily (older women: 1,500–2,000 mg).
- Carotenoids: 10,000–20,000 IU daily.
- Omega-3 fatty acids (fish oil capsules): 50 mg, one to three times daily.
- Potassium: 99 mg, one to three times daily.
- Selenium: 100–200 mcg daily.
- Vitamin A: 5,000–10,000 IU daily.
- Vitamin D: 200–800 IU daily.
- Vitamin E: 400–500 IU daily.

HERBS

- Alfalfa: as directed on label.
- Ginger extract (EV EXT 77): one to two 170-mg capsules daily.
- Ginkgo biloba extract: 60 mg, one to three times daily.
- Rutin: 50 mg, one to three times daily.
- Tarragon oil: as directed on label.
- Turmeric: as directed on label.

TRY

- Eat more cruciferous vegetables.
- Exercise regularly.

AVOID / WATCH OUT FOR

- Alcohol consumption.
- Excess weight.
- High blood pressure.
- Salt and sugar.
- Smoking.
- Stress.

Sunburn

Sunburn results from an overexposure to ultraviolet (UV) rays. Depending on the amount of sun exposure and type of skin pigment a person has, the skin becomes red, swollen, and painful. Later, blisters may form, and the skin may peel. Staying out of strong, direct sunlight is the most obvious and effective way to prevent sunburn. When exposed to the sun, the use of sunscreen is highly recommended. Natural remedies can help speed recovery and reduce the chance of permanent damage.

SUPPLEMENTS

- Potassium: 99 mg, one to three times daily.
- Vitamin C: 500–1,000 mg daily.
- Vitamin E: 400–500 IU daily.

HERBS

- Aloe vera gel: apply topically as directed on label.
- Arnica lotion: apply topically as directed on label.
- Calendula ointment: apply topically as directed on label.
- Chamomile tea: apply topically in compresses.

TRY

- Drink lots of fluids.
- Rub MSM lotion on affected skin.
- Wear sunglasses, sun hat, and loose clothing.

AVOID / WATCH OUT FOR

- Excessive exposure to the sun.
- Retin-A and tetracycline (otherwise, when taking these drugs, avoid excessive exposure to the sun).

Surgery

If you are facing surgery, chances are you want to do all you can to make sure you are in tip-top condition. After surgery, you will want to recover as soon as possible. Certain nutritional supplements and herbs can help bring your body to peak condition before surgery, and can help return your body to a healthy state afterward. Be sure to let your surgeon know that you are taking supplements. Find out how long before the scheduled surgery you should stop taking them and when would be a good time to resume using them.

SURGERY

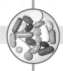

SUPPLEMENTS

- Coenzyme Q_{10}: 60 mg, one to three times daily.
- Vitamin A: 5,000–10,000 IU daily.
- Vitamin C: 500–1,000 mg daily.
- Vitamin E: 400–500 IU daily.
- Zinc: 15 mg of elemental zinc (read label), once or twice daily.

HERBS

- Ginseng tea: drink one cup daily.
- Grape seed/green tea complex: 100 mg of each twice daily.
- Kava: as directed on label.
- Licorice root: one to three 450-mg capsules daily.
- Milk thistle (silymarin) capsules: 140 mg, one to three times daily.
- St. John's wort/phenol complex (for anxiety): 300 mg, once or twice daily.
- White willow bark (for pain): one to two 500-mg capsules, two to three times daily.
- *See caution under "Avoid / Watch Out For" below.*

TRY

- Drink lots of fluids after surgery.
- Eat more fiber-rich foods.

AVOID / WATCH OUT FOR

- Alcohol for forty-eight hours before and after surgery.
- Herbs for forty-eight hours after surgery; check with your surgeon before resuming.
- Highly processed foods.
- Refined sugar and food additives.

Taste Loss

Taste loss is rarely ever a life-threatening condition, but it certainly takes away from the enjoyment of sitting down to a delicious meal. The senses of taste and smell are closely linked. If you cannot smell your food, as in the case of a stuffed nose, your sense of taste will be diminished. This is usually a temporary condition. Loss of taste can also result from smoking, as a side effect of prescription medications, or from burns to the taste buds. Natural remedies, especially supplementing with zinc, can restore taste to make eating the enjoyable experience it should be.

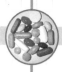

SUPPLEMENTS

- Multivitamin/mineral/antioxidant formula: as directed on label.
- Zinc: 15 mg of elemental zinc (read label), once or twice daily.

HERBS

- No herbs apply.

TRY

- Saltwater nasal drops.

Toothache

Anyone who has had a toothache knows just how painful and annoying they can be. A toothache may result from a cavity, an abscess, inflammation of the gum around the root of the tooth, or sinus inflammation. In cases of very painful toothaches, immediate attention by a dentist is very important. For milder toothaches and to prevent them from occurring, a number of natural remedies can be highly effective. However, even in the case of mild toothaches, make an appointment to see your dentist. See also SINUSITIS.

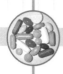

SUPPLEMENTS

- Calcium: 500–1,000 mg daily (older women: 1,500–2,000 mg).
- Coenzyme Q_{10}: 60 mg, one to three times daily.
- Folic acid: 400–800 mg daily.
- Vitamin C: 500–1,000 mg daily with 500 mg of bioflavonoids daily.
- Vitamin D: 200–800 IU daily.

HERBS

- Evening primrose oil capsules: 500–1,000 mg daily.
- Green tea extract: 100 mg tablets, twice daily, or drink one to two cups of tea daily.
- Oil of cloves: apply to affected area with a toothpick.

TRY

- Bite chili peppers.
- Brush carefully.
- Use a gum stimulator.

AVOID / WATCH OUT FOR

- Dried fruits.
- High-carbohydrate foods.
- Potato chips.
- Sipping sugared beverages.

Toxicity

TOXICITY

There are many toxins, or poisons, in our
environment—bacteria, fumes, heavy metals,
drugs, and so on—that can all contribute to an
overall toxic condition. This toxic condition can
contribute to, or aggravate, many other ailments
discussed in this book. A good detoxification
program, such as the one suggested on the
facing page, can not only help you feel better
overall, but can also help clear up stubborn
symptoms attributed to other causes.

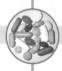

SUPPLEMENTS

- Fiber: 6–12 grams daily.
- Glutamine: 50–150 mg daily.
- MSM: 1,000 mg, one to three times daily.
- Multi–trace mineral formula: as directed on label.

HERBS

- Burdock root: as directed on label.
- Cascara sagrada: as directed on label.
- Dandelion: as directed on label.
- Echinacea: as directed on label.
- Goldenseal: as directed on label.
- Licorice root: one to three 450-mg capsules daily.
- Milk thistle (silymarin) capsules: 140 mg, one to three times daily.
- Oregon grape root: as directed on label.
- Parsley: as directed on label.
- Uva ursi: as directed on label.
- Yellow dock: as directed on label.

TRY

- A professional high colonic enema.
- Drink six to eight glasses of pure water daily.
- Eat more fiber-rich foods.
- Sit in a sauna once daily.

AVOID / WATCH OUT FOR

- Environmental toxins/pollution.
- Excess alcohol consumption.
- Junk food.

Ulcer, Peptic

A peptic ulcer is a well-defined round sore where the lining of the stomach has been eaten away by stomach acid and digestive juices. It usually develops when the defense mechanisms protecting the stomach from acid break down. Ulcer symptoms—gnawing, soreness, and burning in the stomach—tend to occur when the stomach is empty and often come and go as the day wears on. While most people turn to antacids and other such medicines to relieve them of ulcers, many natural therapies can be just as effective and are usually safer.

SUPPLEMENTS

- Betaine hydrochloride (HCL): one 150-mg capsule with each meal.
- Digestive enzymes: one to three capsules with each meal.
- Glutamine 50–150 mg daily.
- Pectin: 500–1,500 mg daily.
- Vitamin E: 400–500 IU daily.

HERBS

- Aloe vera juice: one tablespoon twice daily.
- Cabbage juice: one tablespoon two to three times daily.
- Cayenne: as directed on label.
- Licorice root: one to three 450-mg capsules daily.
- Papaya tablets (chewable): one to three tablets after a meal or eat the fruit after a large meal.

TRY

- Eat yogurt with live cultures.

AVOID / WATCH OUT FOR

- Animal fats.
- Caffeine, alcohol, and soda.
- Fried foods.
- NSAIDs (nonsteroidal anti-inflammatory drugs).
- Salt and strong spices.

Urinary Tract Infection

The kidneys, bladder, ureters, and urethra comprise the urinary tract. Urinary tract infections are commonly caused by bacteria, but may also be caused by fungi, viruses, or parasites. A common infection of the urinary tract is urethritis—infection of the urethra. Symptoms include pain during urination and a frequent urge to urinate. This condition is often treated with antibiotics; however, it is possible to treat it naturally and prevent it from occurring by incorporating simple steps into your daily routine. See also CYSTITIS.

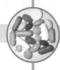

SUPPLEMENTS

- Magnesium: 250–500 mg daily.
- Vitamin A: 5,000–10,000 IU daily.
- Vitamin B_6 (pyridoxine): 25–50 mg daily.
- Vitamin C: 500–1,000 mg daily.

HERBS

- Cranberry juice extract: as directed on label.
- Marshmallow root: as directed on label.
- Oregon grape root: as directed on label.
- Uva ursi: as directed on label.

TRY

- Acupuncture.
- Always wipe front to back.
- Drink six to eight glasses of pure water daily.
- Drink two 8-ounce glasses of unsweetened cranberry juice daily.
- Homeopathic bladder infection remedy.
- Take a sitz bath.
- Urinate when you feel the urge and immediately after intercourse.

AVOID / WATCH OUT FOR

- Holding urine.
- Tight-fitting clothing.
- Wiping back to front.

Vaginal Dryness

One of the primary symptoms of menopause, vaginal dryness leads to irritation, inflammation, itching, and tenderness of the vagina. Continued dryness sometimes leads to yeast infections and vaginitis. Vaginal dryness is not something that should be simply accepted as an inevitable consequence of menopause. There are quite a few natural methods that can be used to help alleviate the problem. See also MENOPAUSE.

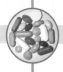

SUPPLEMENTS

- None apply.

HERBS

- Dong quai: as directed on label.
- Vitex (chasteberry): as directed on label.

TRY

- Eat more protein.
- Natural progesterone cream (if that does not work, try a small amount of natural estrogen cream).

AVOID / WATCH OUT FOR

- Excess weight.
- Overexercising.
- Stress.
- Synthetic hormones (HRT).

Vaginal Yeast Infection

A yeast infection (candidiasis) is a very common infection of the vagina that causes discharge, itching, and swelling. It is caused by a fungus called *Candida,* which lives in the body all the time but occasionally gets out of control. People with diabetes and pregnant women are particularly prone to this infection. It is not serious and can often be relieved with the help of natural remedies. See also CANDIDIASIS.

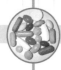

SUPPLEMENTS

- Acidophilus: one to three (multi-billion count) capsules before each meal.
- Caprylic acid supplement: one to three times daily.
- Garlic: 500 mg daily.
- MSM: 1,000 mg, one to three times daily.
- Shitake mushroom extract: as directed on label.

HERBS

- Barberry: as directed on label.
- Chamomile: as directed on label.
- Cinnamon: as directed on label.
- Dandelion: as directed on label.
- Echinacea: as directed on label.
- Licorice root: one to three 450-mg capsules daily.
- Pau d'arco: as directed on label.

TRY

- Boric acid solution douche.
- Eat raw garlic.
- Eat shitake mushrooms.
- Tea tree oil douche.

AVOID / WATCH OUT FOR

- Simple carbohydrates.
- Yeast-containing foods.

Varicose Veins

Varicose veins, which usually occur in the legs, are bluish, swollen, stretched veins that can often be seen bulging through the skin. This condition sometimes causes discomfort and aching in the legs, especially when it is first beginning to develop. Thought to be due in part to heredity, varicose veins cannot be reversed. Surgery to remove as many of the veins as possible is sometimes undertaken. However, natural steps can be taken to improve the appearance of the veins, reduce the associated discomfort, and possibly reduce the chances of more developing.

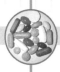

SUPPLEMENTS

- Bioflavonoids: 500 mg daily to strengthen capillaries.
- Vitamin E: 400–500 IU daily.

HERBS

- Buckthorn: as directed on label.
- Butcher's broom: as directed on label.
- Cascara sagrada: as directed on label.
- Ginkgo biloba extract: 60 mg, one to three times daily.
- Gotu kola: as directed on label.

TRY

- Detoxification (see TOXICITY on page 186).
- Eat more fiber for bowel movements.
- Eat more fruits and vegetables.
- Exercise regularly, including stretching.
- Yoga.

AVOID / WATCH OUT FOR

- High-fat diet.
- Hot, spicy foods.
- Sitting for long periods.
- Straining during bowel movements.

Vertigo

People with vertigo have the uncomfortable sensation that either they or the objects around them are spinning or moving. This is often accompanied by a loss of balance and feelings of nausea. Vertigo, which can last from several hours to a few days, has several causes, the most common of which is motion sickness. Motion sickness itself results from heightened sensitivity of the inner ear to movement. Natural remedies can help prevent a bout with vertigo as well as help reduce the unsettling feeling once it's occurred.

SUPPLEMENTS

- Calcium: 500–1,000 mg daily (older women: 1,500–2,000 mg).
- Vitamin B_6 (pyridoxine): 25–50 mg daily.

HERBS

- Ginger root extract: as directed on label.
- Ginkgo biloba extract: 60 mg, one to three times daily.

TRY

- Acupuncture.
- Low-salt diet.

AVOID / WATCH OUT FOR

- Amusement-park rides.
- Boating.
- Glass elevators in high-rise buildings.

Vision Problems

As people age, visual acuity, or clarity of vision, tends to decrease, and vision becomes blurry. Many consider this an inevitable effect of advancing age. Middle-aged people often discover that their eyesight "isn't what it used to be." However, your eyesight doesn't "have to go" just because you're getting older. In addition to regularly seeing an ophthalmologist, taking natural steps now can protect your vision later in life. See also CATARACTS.

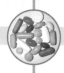

SUPPLEMENTS

- N-acetylcysteine: 1,500 mg with meals.
- Selenium: 100–200 mcg daily.
- Vitamin A: 5,000–10,000 IU daily.
- Vitamin C: 500–1,000 mg daily.
- Vitamin E: 400–500 IU daily.

HERBS

- Bilberry extract: as directed on label.
- Evening primrose oil capsules: 500–1,000 mg daily.
- Ginkgo biloba extract: 60 mg, one to three times daily.
- Grape seed extract (PCOs): 100 mg, one to three times daily.
- Quercetin: 400 mg before eating, one to three times daily.

TRY

- Eat fish rich in omega-3 fatty acids.
- Eat green, orange, and yellow vegetables.

AVOID / WATCH OUT FOR

- Excess sugar consumption.
- Hydrogenated oils.
- Prescription drugs.

Wounds

A wound is defined as a break in the structure
of an organ or tissue caused by an external
agent. Put simply, if you've ever been bruised,
grazed, cut, punctured, or burned, you've
received a wound. Wounds are treated in a
variety of ways, depending on severity and
type. There are many natural remedies that can
be very effective in helping to heal wounds
more quickly.

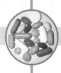

SUPPLEMENTS

- Bromelain: as directed on label.
- Vitamin C: 500–1,000 mg daily.
- Vitamin E: 400–500 IU daily.
- Zinc: 15 mg of elemental zinc (read label), once or twice daily.

HERBS

- Aloe vera gel: apply topically as directed on label.
- Calendula ointment or gel: apply topically as directed on label.
- Comfrey tea: apply topically.

TRY

- Vitamin E cream.
- Wash with antibacterial soap and water.

AVOID / WATCH OUT FOR

- Aspirin and other blood-thinners.

Wrinkles

Wrinkles are usually thought of as one the first signs of aging. As we age, our skin becomes less firm, resulting in some creases and lines that are ultimately unavoidable. The number of wrinkles we develop and the severity of them, however, can be controlled. The best thing that can be done to protect your skin from wrinkles is to avoid excessive exposure to sunlight as much as possible. Beyond that, there are a number of natural methods and remedies that can be used to both help protect and restore vitality to your skin.

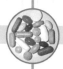

SUPPLEMENTS

- DHEA: 25 mg daily for women over forty; 50 mg daily for men over forty.
- Multivitamin/mineral/antioxidant formula: as directed on label.
- Nucleic Acids (RNA and DNA): 100–300 mg daily.
- SOD (Superoxidedismutase): 125 mcg daily.
- Vitamin C: 500–1,000 mg daily.
- Vitamin E: 400–500 IU daily.

HERBS

- Wild yam: as directed on label.

TRY

- Drink six to ten glasses of pure water daily.
- Eat fresh fruits and vegetables.
- Get enough sleep (at least seven to eight hours).
- Lose weight if necessary.

AVOID / WATCH OUT FOR

- Excessive sun exposure.

Therapies

ACUPUNCTURE/ACUPRESSURE

Acupuncture is a practice that originated in China in which tiny needles are inserted at specific points on the body to relieve pain and cure disease. In acupressure, the practitioner applies pressure to the specific sites instead of inserting needles into the skin. When performed by a qualified practitioner, both of these methods can produce positive results. Many people report a reduction in pain and symptoms—and sometimes, complete relief.

ALLERGY ELIMINATION DIET

In an allergy elimination diet, you remove all suspect foods from your diet for two weeks. Suspect foods may include dairy, wheat, shellfish, and gluten. If no improvement is seen, you may still be eating foods that you are allergic to. Try to eliminate as many more foods as possible. When you are no longer experiencing any symptoms, add one eliminated food back to your diet. (Of course, if you know for sure that you are allergic to it, do not add it back.) If there is no reaction after two to three hours, that particular food should be safe to eat. Then, each week, add one more food back to your diet. This way, you should be able to determine which foods are causing the problem. Once you know which they are, be sure not to eat them at all or symptoms may return.

AROMATHERAPY

Aromatherapy is the practice of using essential oils—the distilled essences of plants, fruits, and flowers—to promote and enhance physical and emotional well-being. Essential oils can be inhaled from the bottle, applied to the skin in carrier oils, added to bathwater, used in therapeutic steam inhalations, and dispersed in the air with a diffuser. It's important to purchase essential oils from a reputable manufacturer to make sure that the products you buy are pure. Also, when purchasing aromatherapy products, such as candles, be sure that they actually contain essential oils and no synthetic fragrances.

BIOFEEDBACK

Biofeedback is a treatment technique in which a person receives immediate feedback on unconscious or involuntary body processes to eventually gain control over them. Clinical biofeedback is often used successfully for pain management, muscle movement and control, and circulatory dysfunction. If you think biofeedback might help your condition, seek out a trained biofeedback therapist in your area. Depending on your needs, the therapist may recommend a course of several sessions in addition to at-home practice.

DOUCHING

A douche is a preparation of water usually mixed with a healing substance that is jetted into the vagina using a special device. Commonly used to simply cleanse the vagina, douches can also be used for healing purposes. Store-bought douches often contain harsh chemicals and should be avoided. You can purchase a device specifically for douching at your pharmacy and can prepare a natural solution at home, using vinegar and water, unprocessed plain yogurt with live cultures, boric acid and water, or a few drops of tea tree oil and water. Douche only occasionally, as frequent douching can upset the balance of healthy bacteria normally present in the vagina.

EXERCISE

Exercise

Exercise is important for a healthy body, but many people do not get enough regular exercise. A strong, toned body is less susceptible to infections and recovers quicker. Exercise also relieves stress, which strengthens the immune system. When regular exercise is recommended, it doesn't necessarily mean that you should run laps or lift heavy weights. Exercise can simply be taking a long walk, climbing stairs, participating in a sport, or any number of other physical daily activities. If you haven't exercised for a long time, start slowly and increase your activity when you feel you can handle it. Before starting any type of exercise program, check with your doctor.

FRESH FRUIT DIET

If you are suffering from a weakened immune system, a temporary diet consisting of fresh fruit can help to strengthen it. While on this diet, you eat only fresh fruit for two to three days. You can also juice the fruit occasionally, but the fiber that you get from the whole fruit is important. Dark-colored fruits are best, and although they are not fruits, dark green leafy vegetables are also good to eat. While you are on this diet, you can continue taking your regular supplements. Be sure to drink six to ten glasses of water daily while on this diet to prevent changes in your bowel movements. When you go off this diet, you should add other foods back in slowly.

HOMEOPATHY

Homeopathy is a time-tested practice of treating a disorder by administering small doses of a remedy that would produce the symptoms of that disorder in a healthy person. Homeopathy has become a well-respected alternative to conventional medicine. Homeopathic remedies for virtually everything from acne to warts can be found on the shelves of nutrition centers and health food stores. Moreover, homeopathic practitioners who tailor remedies to your specific needs are becoming increasingly more common.

MASSAGE

Massage

Body massage can be described as the manipulation of soft tissue for therapeutic purposes. Massages can successfully treat illnesses brought about by stress, such as tension, aches and pains, insomnia, and headaches, all of which are accumulated in the course of daily life. The pain-relieving effects associated with skin stimulation and increased temperature that result from a massage help induce relaxation, both mentally and physically. It is very popular today to regularly attend a spa, where any number of different massages from shiatsu to Swedish are available. However, trading massages with a partner or friend is less costly.

MEDITATION

Meditation

Meditation is the practice of sitting calmly and emptying one's mind of day-to-day concerns and concentrating on one specific thought or *mantra,* a word or phrase that embodies an ideal or guiding principle. When practiced regularly—for anywhere from five minutes to a half-hour each day—meditation can help induce relaxation and promote clearer thinking. Meditation centers are becoming more common, but you can meditate anywhere—even on a long line at the bank. Also, guided meditation audio tapes are widely available.

SAUNAS

Saunas

A sauna is a steam bath in which water is poured on hot coals to produce steam. Many gyms, health spas, and resorts have a room specifically for this purpose. Some people even have them installed in their homes—usually at a great expense. The temperature in these rooms can be quite high, so anyone who is ill should avoid them or discuss their use with a doctor. In relatively healthy people, saunas promote relaxation and help cleanse the body of toxins because the humidity and high temperatures promote sweating. The time spent in the sauna should be limited to about ten to twenty minutes, and should be followed by a shower.

TAI CHI

Tai Chi

Developed in ancient China, tai chi is a type of meditative exercise. In this system, a series of preset movements are performed slowly and fluidly. While practitioners may make it look easy, it does require quite a bit of effort. The benefit is that it has an overall relaxing effect on the body and mind. Centers that have tai chi classes are becoming more common. Some martial arts studios and health clubs may also offer tai chi classes. While it's a good idea to learn the techniques from an instructor, tai chi videotapes are available so that you can practice in your own home.

YOGA

Yoga is a system of poses that developed in ancient India. It induces relaxation and improves the flexibility of your muscles. Presently, there are many different styles of yoga. If you are interested in this system, it's a good idea to research what types of yoga are available in your area and determine which is right for you. While certain philosophies are often attached to this practice, it can be performed without this connection. Many health clubs and centers offer daily yoga classes. Once you learn the poses, you can easily practice at home.

About
the Author

Earl Mindell, R.Ph., Ph.D., is an internationally recognized expert on nutrition, drugs, vitamins, and herbal remedies. He is the author of forty-five books, including the *Vitamin Bible for the 21st Century, Prescription Alternatives, Soy Miracle, New Herb Bible, Anti-Aging Bible, Peak Performance Bible,* and *The Diet Bible.* He is a registered pharmacist, master herbalist, and a professor of nutrition at Pacific Western University in Los Angeles. He conducts nutritional seminars around the world and lives in Beverly Hills, California.